HEINERMAN'S
Encyclopedia of

JUICES
TEAS &
TONICS

D1214936

OTHER BOOKS BY
THE SAME AUTHOR

HEINERMAN'S
Encyclopedia of
JUICES
TEAS &
TONICS

John Heinerman

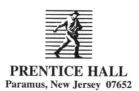

PRENTICE HALL
Paramus, New Jersey 07652

Library of Congress Cataloging-in-Publication Data

Heinerman, John.
   [Encyclopedia of juices, teas, & tonics]
   Heinerman's encyclopedia of juices, teas, & tonics / John
Heinerman.
      p. cm.
   Includes index.
   ISBN 0-13-234204-9 (C)—ISBN 0-13-234196-4 (P)
    1. Fruit juices—Therapeutic use—Encyclopedias. 2. Vegetable
juices—Therapeutic use—Encyclopedias. 3. Herbal teas—Therapeutic
use—Encyclopedias. 4. Tonics (Medicinal preparations)—
Encyclopedias I. Title.
RM255.H447 1996   96-33721
615'.32—dc20   CIP

Printed in the United States of America

10 9 8 7 6 5 4 3 2 (C)   10 9 8 7 6 5 4 3 (P)

ISBN 0-13-234204-9 (C)   ISBN 0-13-234196-4 (P)

PRENTICE HALL
Paramus, NJ 07652

A Simon & Schuster Company

On the World Wide Web at http://www.phdirect.com

Prentice-Hall International (UK) Limited, *London*
Prentice-Hall of Australia Pty. Limited, *Sydney*
Prentice-Hall Canada Inc., *Toronto*
Prentice-Hall Hispanoamericana, S.A., *Mexico*
Prentice-Hall of India Private Limited, *New Delhi*
Prentice-Hall of Japan, Inc., *Tokyo*
Simon & Schuster Asia Pte. Ltd., *Singapore*
Editora Prentice-Hall do Brasil, Ltda., *Rio de Janeiro*

To

C. Allen Huntington, George W. Grant, and David P. Kimball, three 18-year-old Mormon pioneer boys, who in the bitter winter of 1856 put their own lives in jeopardy to single-handedly rescue the survivors of the ill-fated Martin handcart company who were close to death themselves in the mountains of Wyoming. Their noble acts of heroism made Mormon Church leader Brigham Young weep like a child when he heard of it. All three died a few years later in early manhood as a result of the terrible health effects they suffered for their heroism, due to excessive physical strain and weather exposure.

INTRODUCTION

When one of my previous books on the same subject came out two years ago, it took everyone at my publishing house, as well as myself, by surprise. *Heinerman's Encyclopedia of Healing Juices* started out of the gate like the winning race horse that it has become in a burst of speed that left other health titles in the dust.

Now comes this title on the same subject of juices, but also with herbal teas and tonics included. It is intended to be a reliable source of much self-help health information as the other one was. However, I didn't want to have a clone of the first, so I deliberately put together a volume that differs from the previous book in a number of ways.

For one thing, the alphabetized contents are listed by health disorder instead of by juice, tea, or tonic. Another thing quite unique to this work is that toward the end of nearly every entry are given recipe instructions for making the individual juices, teas, or tonics mentioned in each section. This layout uses fewer words and presents the methods of preparation more succinctly than the other book did. Those who have seen this arrangement have pronounced it more clear and concise. As one middle-aged rabbi's wife in the old but upscale section of Squirrel Hill on the outskirts of Pittsburgh told me after being sent a portion of the manuscript to review, "I didn't have to work my way through so much explanation in figuring out how to make the things you recommend. It was there in plain enough English for me to grasp."

A third change has been the inclusion of what might be called "medicinal spirits"—that is to say, certain fermented liquids of the vine with potential healing properties in them. There are a number of remedies employing the use of certain ales, beers, wines, and fine liqueurs that are occasionally mentioned in different sections of the text. This is not, by any means, to say that I advocate drinking alcoholic substances. But it does suggest that some common sense needs to be used in realizing that some of these beverages have wonderful medicinal benefits when appropriately used in *moderation*. And I believe the key here is "moderation in all things."

Probably the biggest surprise in store for my readers are the stories themselves that appear in this book. I will be the first one to admit that they represent, without doubt, some of the most far-ranging themes that have ever been included in any of my previous works.

This is a book that retired cartoonist Gary Larson would definitely appreciate. For a number of years he drew the piece called *The Far Side* which was serialized in more than 2,000 newspapers around the globe. His world was one filled with the offbeat, the unusual, and, most definitely, the weird. His world was peopled with talking cows dressed in chef outfits that served up McPeople burgers and with life-size mosquitoes reaching for cans of Raid insecticide to spray on tiny humans flying in and out of their dwellings and disturbing their peace of mind.

By far the best cartoon panel Larson ever drew, at least from my perspective as a social scientist, was the one poking fun at anthropologists such as myself. It showed the inside of a grass hut with all the amenities of modern living—TV set, VCR, radio, stereo. electric fan, microwave oven, and so forth. The resident jungle natives were hurriedly scampering about trying to hide all these products of modern technology as one of their number looked through an open window to see two bespectacled scientists dressed in khaki attire and carrying notebooks with them approaching in their direction. The caption below describing the warning the one native was yelling, read: "Anthropologists coming! Quick hide everything!" It was intended to suggest that appearances can sometimes be very deceiving if we're not careful in our discernment of things. Here were anthropologists such as myself coming to visit a supposedly primitive tribe that had access to many of the comforts of modern living. This was Larson's style of satire and his range of versatility.

My own efforts in this book, however, are by far more serious, because matters involving the health and well-being of people are not to be taken lightly. But my reasons for making reference to Mr. Larson is to let readers know that I've included here a wide range of true accounts that sometimes border on the bizarre, the mysterious, the dangerous, and even the inscrutable. For me this has been something of a departure from the contents of my other books. The stories in them had been pretty much middle-of-the-road and fairly conservative in nature. But not so in this book. The basic formulas themselves remain the same in terms of tried-and-true effectiveness and producing the results that readers expect. But in terms of story content, be prepared for a tour of reading that is *most definitely* a mind-walk on *The Far Side*.

Consider these few selections taken at random from the pages of this book:

- The Federal Express courier who had a James Bond-type submachine gun stolen from the back of his delivery van and needed some chamomile tea to calm him down.

- The pioneer woman who almost died from fright when she thought a dead corpse was making sounds as if it were coming back to life again; an herb tea helped her to regain her sanity.

- A supernatural experience given to a nationally recognized herbal authority (since deceased) that resulted in a natural remedy that has saved thousand of people's lives who previously suffered from asthma or bronchitis.

- The herbs that could have helped former U.S. Vice-President Dan Quayle with his own life-threatening situation.

- An amazing vegetable ointment for severe skin burns that was developed by a fellow who handles dangerous snakes and drinks poisons like strychnine on a *regular* basis for religious purposes.

- Cures for cancer that really work from one of the most eccentric people ever to appear on the American holistic health scene.

- A very effective cold and flu remedy from a female skydiver who gets her own thrills from 4,000 feet up in the air.

- An old Army remedy to stop diarrhea that was once used by the world's greatest blues musician.

- A secret "surefire" remedy for a major lung disease from a cattle rancher with a true deer hunting tale that is so far out it will knock your socks off with disbelief.

- A widespread "career woman's disease" treated with natural substances that were given to me by a geneticist who is engaged in grafting human ears on the backs of specially bred laboratory mice.

- A liquid tonic for a number of women's problems that is routinely prescribed by several Irish hospitals but manufactured by the same people responsible for producing the renowned *Guinness Book of World Records*.

- The unique tea blend that one female mortician regularly drinks to alleviate her fear of ghosts.

- An amazing jungle remedy that one ruthless South American ex-dictator has used to cure himself of urinary tract infection.

■ A country doctor's soup tonic for getting rid of the unseen "critters" inside us.

This gives you a pretty good idea of the types of stories contained in this book. Many of them are unlike anything you've ever read before in any popular health book. But more amazing than the incredible accounts themselves is the fact that every single one of them *is factual and true!* And, besides this, the remedies mentioned in great detail are very, very effective and will astonish you at just how well they work in most cases!

So, if you've become one of my several million fans from previous writings, then you're certainly in for a treat here. I *guarantee* that you won't be one bit disappointed with the purchase you've made. It will be worth every dollar you've spent. And, most likely, it'll be your *best health investment* in years. So, kick back and sit a spell with a cup of warm herb tea or a nice glass of juice and enjoy the book. It will be the best reading adventure you've had in a while and will literally take you to *The Far Side* of good health.

With love and appreciation for your loyalty and devotion, I remain your friend and benefactor in matters of health forever,

John Heinerman
POB 11471
Salt Lake City, UT 84147
Spring of 1996

CONTENTS

ANGER

ANGINA

ANOREXIA (see Anxiety, Bulimia, and Underweight)

ANXIETY

ARTERIOSCLEROSIS/ATHEROSCLEROSIS

ARTHRITIS

ASTHMA/BRONCHITIS

BACK STRAIN

BAD BREATH/BODY ODOR

BALDNESS

BENIGN PROSTATIC HYPERTROPHY (BPH) (see under Prostate Problems)

BLADDER INFECTION

BLOOD CLOTS

BREAST CANCER

BREAST CYSTS

BREAST TENDERNESS

BREECH BIRTH

BULIMIA

BURNS

CANCER

CANDIDIASIS (see Vaginitis and Yeast Infection)

CATARACTS

CRAMPS

CROHN'S DISEASE

CRYING (UNCONTROLLABLE)

CYSTITIS (see Bladder Infection)

DEPRESSION (see Anxiety, Insomnia, and Mood Swings)

DIABETES

DERMATITIS (see Eczema)

DIARRHEA

DIGESTIVE DISTURBANCES
(see Heartburn, Indigestion, Peptic Ulcer)

DIVERTICULITIS

DYSENTERY

DYSFUNCTIONAL UTERINE BLEEDING

DYSMENORRHEA (see Cramps and Menstrual Difficulties)

GOUT
An Old Russian Cossack Remedy for Uric Acid Accumulations . .

HEADACHE
Herbal Tea Secrets from the Tenth Annual Conference of the International Herb Association . . . .

HEARTBURN
Fruit Juices and Herb Teas to Soothe Burning Sensations . . . . . .

HEART DISEASE
Elixirs for Preventing Diseases of the Heart and Liver . . . .

HEMORRHOIDS
Iced Tea Compress and Green Chlorophyll for Treating Piles . . .

HERPES ZOSTER
Oatmeal Water and Spinach Juice Work Unbelievable Wonders . .

HIATAL HERNIA (see Heartburn)

HIGH BLOOD PRESSURE
Hot Vegetable Tonic for Normalizing Blood Pressure . . . .

HOT FLASHES
Cooling Herbal Beverages from the Orient for Flushes . . . .

HUMAN PAPILLOMA
Grape Juice Strengthens the Immune System to Fight HP Virus . . .

HYPERTENSION (see High Blood Pressure)

HYPOGLYCEMIA (see Mood Swings)

HYPOTHERMIA
Tomato Zinger for Raising Internal Body Temperature . . . .

WARTS

WORMS

YEAST INFECTION

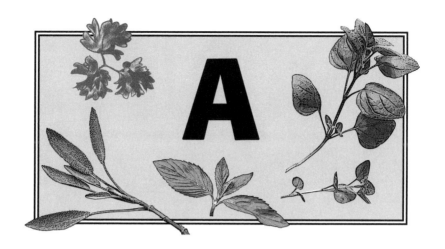

ACNE

Clear Skin Again with Red Clover Tea

DESCRIPTION

Red clover occurs most often in meadows, cleared fields, pastures, and along roadsides everywhere. It was first introduced from Europe several centuries ago, but eventually became naturalized throughout much of Canada and the United States.

Red clover is a short-lived perennial capable of growing almost a yard in height. It appears in clumps that consist of several smooth or hairy stems. The green leaves are stalked and have three oval leaflets, each one usually carrying the trademark whitish V-shaped marking. The flowerheads appear from spring to fall, are round and an inch in width, and vary from pink to rose in hue.

High School Cheerleader Enjoys Clear Complexion

A member of my staff has a 17-year-old daughter who attends a local high school in Salt Lake City. Tamara is a very popular girl in school with the guys—she's the cheerleader whom many of them fight over to see who gets the first date with her.

One would think that this would make any girl feel as if she were in "seventh heaven." But a while ago Tamara was quite unhappy, not so much with her enviable situation at school, but rather with her complexion. You see, Tamara suffered from whiteheads and blackheads. This made her very self-conscious. Her mom informed me that her girl even lost some of her self-esteem because of this.

Since she knew I was an authority on medicinal plants, she asked what herb might be helpful for her daughter's unhappy situation. Knowing that red clover is terrific for skin problems, I immediately recommended this.

My staff assistant went to the health food store and bought a box of cut, dried red clover blossoms. She went home and made a tea according to my instructions. Bring 1 quart of distilled or spring water almost to the boiling point. Then add 3/4 cup red clover blossoms. Stir thoroughly, cover with a lid, and set aside to steep for 40 minutes. Strain and store in the refrigerator.

On my suggestion, Tamara began washing her face with bar soap containing wheat germ and oatmeal. Afterwards, she rinsed with regular water and then *rinsed a second time* with some of this red clover tea. She also drank one small glass of the tea twice daily between meals. In addition to this, she also cut out of her diet anything that was greasy or sugary.

Within two weeks her complexion cleared up and she once again regained total confidence in herself. She attributed her improved image appearance to the red clover tea and good diet.

Skin Cancer Stopped

In one of my other encyclopedic works having to do with plants (*Heinerman's Encyclopedia of Healing Herbs and Spices* [Englewood Cliffs, NJ: Prentice Hall, 1995]), I discuss at length under the entry for RED CLOVER the different medical benefits to be obtained from using this tea *consistently* in the treatment of cancer.

I cited a true account of one particular gentleman in the nineteenth century who suffered from a recurring case of melanoma for some years. He had consulted with a number of prominent physicians of his day, none of whom seemed to have offered him much help.

He had almost resigned himself to continued pain and an eventual miserable death when he heard about red clover from someone. He made a tea and both drank it as well as washed the cancerous area around his eye with it on a daily basis. Within a short time, the cancer miraculously disappeared and never came back.

New flesh grew over the area previously damaged by cancer. The man gained weight and experienced increased appetite. He both looked and felt better than he had done in years, much to the amazement of everyone around him who knew of his former sick condition.

Woman Recovers with Tea from Beating

I was over to the house of a friend recently, visiting with him and his wife. Both are of Mexican origin. While there, I met his sister and her two young children. They had been staying for a few nights at the local YWCA women's shelter because of her ex-husband.

It seems that he had been taking crack (an illicit drug made from cocaine), which often put him in a foul mood. He and this woman got into a fierce argument, which ultimately led to a bad beating for her. When I saw her for the first time, she had ugly bruises on her face, neck, arms, back, and legs.

She wanted to know if there was anything that could be done to minimize the bruises, since she had to go back to work as a checker in a local supermarket the following week. I recommended red clover tea and a homeopathic remedy of arnica tincture for this.

Because none of these people were well acquainted with a health food store, I purchased for her the things she needed, for which I was reimbursed. I showed her how to make some red clover tea according to instructions previously given in this section. But the tea was steeped for only 20 minutes, strained, and then divided into two parts. One part was refrigerated until it became quite cold and the other part reheated until it was somewhat hot.

I got two white terry washcloths and a pair of small hand towels. I showed my friend, his wife, and his sister what to do next. With a pair of ice tongs, I immersed one washcloth in the hot water, lifted it out, and squeezed out the excess liquid with one hand. I wore a pair of plastic gloves so as not to burn myself. This I then folded in half and placed over a large, ugly, purple swelling and covered it with one of the dry towels to retain the heat better.

After it became cool, I removed it and placed on it the other folded washcloth, which had been soaked in the cold water and wrung out. I covered it also with the hand towel to hold in the coolness longer. I told her she was to do this for half an hour twice a day on the worst of her bruises for three days.

After each application she was to apply some of the arnica tincture on every spot being treated. Larger areas were covered with a folded layer of gauze soaked with some of this tincture and held in place with tape. For smaller bruises, though, I told her just to put some drops of liquid arnica in the middle of a Band-Aid, then place it over the skin and leave it there for 24 hours before changing it again.

By the end of five days nearly all the terrible discolorations had disappeared and she seemed to feel a lot better about herself as the result of this treatment.

COMPLEXION TEA

Here's my own original recipe for making yourself a tea that will do wonders for your skin.

1 pint distilled water

¹/₄ cup red clover blossoms

1 tbsp. dried rose hips

1 tsp. shredded lemon peel

1 tsp. peppermint leaves

Boil the water in a stainless steel, enamel, or glass pot. *Do not use aluminum for this.* Add the rose hips and lemon peel. Cover with a lid and gently simmer for 5 minutes.

Uncover and add the red clover and peppermint. Cover again and set aside to steep for 30 minutes. Strain and store in the refrigerator.

Reheat one-half cup as needed. Using cotton balls moistened with some of this tea, scrub the forehead, face, neck, and throat with circular motions morning and evening. You'll be surprised at just how quickly your complexion will become beautiful *and young again!*

AGING

How a 40-Year-Old Who Looked 60 Recovered Her Youthful Appeal

DESCRIPTION

Chlorophyll is the green pigment that gives most plants their color and enables them to carry on a process called photosynthesis. Chemically, chlorophyll has several similar forms, each containing a complex ring structure and a long hydrocarbon tail.

The molecular structure of the chlorophyll is astonishingly similar to that of the heme portion of hemoglobin or red blood in humans. The only exception, however, is that the latter contains iron in place of magnesium. But it would certainly be within the bounds of truth to call chlorophyll "plant *blood*."

Within the photosynthetic cells of plants the chlorophyll is in the chloroplasts—small, roundish, dense protoplasmic bodies that contain the disks where the chlorophyll molecules are found.

Chlorophyll tends to mask the presence of colors in plants from other substances, such as the caretonoids. When the amount of chlorophyll decreases, the other colors become readily apparent. This effect can be seen most dramatically every fall when the leaves of trees "turn color."

The health food industry has turned to various forms of plant life for sources of chlorophyll. These include simple algaes such as chlorella and spirulina, seaweeds such as dulse and kelp, and cereal grasses, primarily wheat and barley.

The sources of good, rich chlorophyll come from wheat and barley grasses grown in the soils of Lawrence, Kansas during the winter months and then harvested at the first jointing stage when the young blades of tender grass appear. Such high-quality chlorophyll is available in juice extracts or tablets from Pines, Inc. (see APPENDIX II under Pines for more information).

How a Schoolteacher Turned Back Her Own "Aging Clock"

One of the most remarkable stories I've shared with my audiences at different health conventions that I routinely speak at concerns the elementary-school teacher from Barstow, California. I'll not use her real name, but instead simply refer to her as Ellen.

I met her three and a half years ago while giving an herb lecture in that city. She came to me with a specific health question and had a young girl by her side. As I looked at Ellen's line-filled face, dull eyes, gray hair, and anemic complexion, I fancied someone almost 60 years of age. Without giving more careful thought to my words, I blurted out, "You have a lovely *grandchild* here."

She took immediate exception to what I had just said and promptly corrected me in a very decisive manner. "That is my *daughter,* I'll have you know," she said icily. I smiled in embarrassment and offered a sincere apology. This warmed her up and she asked, almost with a laugh in her voice, "My goodness, just *how* old do I really look, anyway?" I very softly said, almost timidly, "Uh, would you believe, *sixty?*"

She shook her head in dismay, but didn't get worked up by my response. In fact, to my surprise, she admitted that she *looked* a lot older than she really was. "Even the children in my classroom at the elementary school where I teach," she continued, "will sometimes call me *Grandma* instead of by my last name. Either they do this mistakenly or out of fun."

She then asked with obvious sincerity in her voice, "What can I do to turn back my own 'aging clock'? At this point in time, even a few years will be much appreciated."

I told Ellen about the wonderful benefits of chlorophyll and how this green substance contains many antioxidants that can stop the activity of free radicals within the body. Free radicals, I explained to her, are like tiny molecular sharks zipping around in our cellular seas, taking chemical chomps out of the atoms that make up our muscle tissue, joints, bones, blood, hair, and skin. We get them, I told her, from much of the cooked, processed foods we eat. I noted that hamburgers, for instance, contain more free radicals than any other food I'm aware of, simply because of how they're prepared and cooked.

Because her busy schedule didn't allow her the luxury of juicing dark, leafy greens, I opted to recommend some chlorophyll products from Pines, Inc., that would help to restore some of her lost youthfulness. I furnished her with the address and number of this company (listed in Appendix II) and suggested that she take some of their wheat and barley grass juice extracts each day.

Not liking the direct taste of them, she began mixing 1 teaspoonful of each in 8 fluid ounces of tomato or carrot juice, taking a glass every morning and evening with meals. Later, she discovered that they could also be added to milk or orange juice. She stayed on this regimen for a full two months.

Ellen sent me a color snapshot of herself. At first, I could hardly believe it was the same woman with whom I had talked before. What a change and difference there was between the mental image I had and this photograph. Had I not known better, I would have surely thought they were two different women.

This schoolteacher looked absolutely radiant in the photograph. Most of the tiny crow's feet and wrinkles in her face were almost gone. Her eyes sparkled with life, and she now had a rosy color in her cheeks. Much but not all of her gray hair had disappeared, and she swore in the letter that accompanied it, that she had *not* colored her hair for the photo.

"This is what those two chlorophyll products did for me!" she stated with obvious exuberance. "I was able to turn back my own 'aging clock.' In fact, thanks to those cereal grasses and your own efforts in acquainting me with them, I have regained much of my former youthful appeal." She went on to say, in a teasing way, "Now, some of the young boys in my class come up and kid me about wanting to go out on dates with them. As they're under the age of ten, I seriously doubt their parents would approve of such a thing. But at least it's nice to know I'm thought of as being young and beautiful again."

AGELESS GREEN DRINK

This is a zesty cocktail that has proven of great benefit to those seeking to retain a youthful quality to their complexions. Drinking a glass of this every other day helps to keep the skin from wrinkling so fast and keeps most of the gray out of scalp hair.

$^1/_2$ *cup carrots*

$^1/_3$ *cup celery*

1 large romaine lettuce leaf

$^1/_2$ *handful of cut escarole leaves*

15 parsley sprigs

2 fresh peppermint leaves

$^1/_2$ *cup spinach leaves*

$^3/_4$ *cup canned pineapple juice, chilled*

$^3/_4$ *cup bottled apple juice, chilled*

$1^1/_4$ *cups ice cubes*

Use a Vita-Mix whole-food machine or equivalent blender for making this. Place all the ingredients in the Vita-Mix Total Nutrition Center container in the order given. Secure in place the two-part lid by locking under tabs. Move the black speed control lever to HIGH, then lift the black lever to the ON position.

Run the machine for almost 2 minutes. Makes a little over two cups of dynamic green drink. (See Appendix II for more information on the Vita-Mix unit.)

ALCOHOLISM

Tomato Tonic Saves an Uncle's Liver and Keeps Him Sober

DESCRIPTION

The tomato is related to the potato and eggplant and is a member of the nightshade family. It was cultivated in ancient times from Mexico to Peru by early cultures and today is used on a large global scale as a valuable food resource for over one billion people.

When the Spanish conquistadors brought back seed from Central and South America, the plant was grown only as an ornament; it was then known as the love apple. Until the latter part of the nineteenth century the fruit was commonly regarded as poisonous. Dr. John C. Bennett was one of the first Americans to advocate the medicinal and nutritive virtues of tomatoes. According to the publication *Queen City Heritage* (Summer 1992, p. 38), "Bennett's views were reprinted for decades in medical journals, newspapers, and gardening and agricultural periodicals, not only in the United States, but also in Australia, the United Kindgom, and France."

Technically speaking, the tomato is considered to be a fruit, but it is more commonly assigned to the vegetable category because of its diverse uses.

Favorite Uncle Gets Sober and Has His Liver Saved Too

A family from Pittsburgh came to the National Health Federation convention at the ExpoMart in Monroevill, Pennsylvania, the weekend of June 2–4, 1995. They attended my seminar held Friday morning from 11 A.M. to 12 noon. Later, they accompanied me to the Author's Exhibit space where I and other writers autographed our different volumes for interested buyers.

Mrs. Brodie, the wife, took me aside and told me about a personal problem that a close family member had. Her uncle was a terrible alcoholic, and she wanted to know what could be done to help him. Without using the man's real name, I will, hereafter, refer to him only as Uncle Lushwell.

Mrs. Brodie knew well in advance of seeking my advice that it would take more than just herbs, supplements, or food therapy to help her uncle overcome his unfortunate problem.

But her primary concern seemed to be with the effects that so much alcohol intake had on the man's liver. Having been an LPN (Licensed Practical Nurse) for some years, she had a pretty good understanding of what happens to that particular organ of the body when it is subjected to excessive alcohol.

I sat down and wrote out a specific food program for Uncle Lushwell. I noted, with some irony, "Since your relative's problem is found in a glass, the solution will also come out of a glass."

I pointed out that what was crucial here was for her uncle to get *live liquid foods* into his body as quickly as possible. "Up to now," I continued, "the man has been eating nothing but *dead* foods that have been highly processed or overcooked. Not to mention the *dead* beverages that have been killing him by degrees, too."

I formulated a special "Tomato Tonic" that I knew would be of definite therapeutic value to the man's nearly exhausted liver. I instructed Mrs. Brodie on how to put it together using a food blender of some kind, preferably a Vita-Mix Total Nutrition Center. The recipe for this wonderful juice tonic is found at the end of this section.

I gave her other instructions, including these few items:

- *Avoid* cooked, fried, and deep-fried foods as much as possible. Eat only *live, raw* foods.
- Tone down sugar and sugary foods intake.
- Take 3 capsules dandelion root powder twice daily.
- Take 2 capsules goldenseal root powder once daily.
- Take 2 capsules Kyo-Dophilus from Wakunaga each day with meals.

All of the above are available from health food stores in your area. Or see the Appendix for where to obtain them by mail.

Mrs. Brodie thanked me for my time and rewarded my efforts by purchasing some of my books. Almost two months later I received a phone call in the wee hours of the morning. She was calling to tell me that "after the third day, my uncle didn't need a drink any more." There was some other stuff about Uncle Lushwell's health improving substantially. And a subsequent medical checkup some weeks after drinking my "Tomato Tonic" had shown remarkable regeneration of his liver. I have to admit with some obvious embarrassment and slight regret, though, that due to the early morning hour of her call, I was still half asleep. And, for the life of me, I could not recall later upon awakening everything she had told me. But my tonic worked, she was grateful, and that was all that mattered!

Drug Addiction Resolved

A friend of a friend had a son in his early twenties who was taking crack (an illicit drug derived from cocaine). My help was sought in the matter. I recommended a combination of three things, that have always proven useful in ridding the body, especially the liver, of harmful chemical poisons.

I recommended 2 capsules daily of goldenseal root and 4 capsules of turmeric powder. The first can be bought in any health food store or herb shop. But the second has to be purchased in bulk powder from a supermarket and then put into capsules by hand. The empty gelatin capsules can be bought at any drugstore or local pharmacy. You want to get the 0-size for this. Pull a capsule apart and holding the bigger end between your fingers, poke it into a small pile of turmeric powder until the inside of it is more than full. Then fit the smaller end over the top and push down. After making up a few dozen capsules this way, rub them gently between a clean, dry hand towel or a paper towel to remove excess powder that may cling to the outside. Store the capsules in an empty vitamin or aspirin bottle in the cupboard.

I mentioned to this person that turmeric works best when accompanied *with* tomato juice and so should always be taken when drinking some of my tangy Tomato Tonic. The addict was put on this program for an unspecified period of time. While it didn't totally do away with his drug problem, it had the positive effect of *substantially reducing* his dependency on crack.

HEINERMAN'S TANGY TOMATO TONIC

Put all the following items into a food blender or Vita-Mix whole food machine container in the order given.

> 1–2 cups mineral water
>
> $1/2$ cup ice cubes
>
> 1 tsp. each grapefruit, lemon, and lime juices
>
> 1 tsp. each Teriyaki and Tabasco sauces
>
> $1/4$ tsp. granulated kelp (seaweed)
>
> 1 cup tomatoes, quartered
>
> $1/2$ sweet bell pepper (leave seed core intact)
>
> $1/4$ small white or yellow onion, peeled
>
> 15 parsley sprigs

> **1 small celery stalk with leaves intact, cut up**
>
> **¹/₄ tsp. each of cayenne pepper and turmeric powder**
>
> **1 tsp. each Pines' wheat grass and beet root juice powders**
>
> **3 tbsp. liquid Kyolic Garlic**

Secure the lid beneath the tabs and turn the machine on to HIGH speed and blend for 2 minutes. Drink one cup 3 times daily with meals and refrigerate the rest. You may adjust the flavor according to your individual tastes by adding some sea salt or Mrs. Dash seasoning. The kelp and Kyolic Garlic are found in health food stores; consult the Appendix for Pines' products or call 1-800-MY PINES. Everything else you can get in a supermarket.

ALLERGIES

An Oklahoma Family Spared Symptoms with My Parsley Tonic

DESCRIPTION

Parsley is an aromatic herb that originated in the Mediterranean a long time ago. It is related to the carrot family and has been cultivated since the times of the Roman Empire for its foliage, cookery seasoning, and plate garnish. Also, in ancient times it was used to adorn head wreaths worn by Roman emperors, victorious generals, and illustrious senators. Parsley was sometimes used as a funeral decoration also.

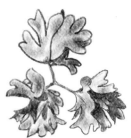

Parsley is widely grown throughout America, especially in Louisiana. It is more often than not ignored by diners in restaurants and constitutes a major plate waste after tables are bussed and utensils sent back into the kitchen to the dishwashers. This is most unfortunate, considering that parsley ranks very high in vitamins A and C, iron, magnesium, calcium, potassium, and phosphorus.

Allergies Alleviated

The following comes as a *true* story from an Oklahoma family. Liz Sherwood of Jones, Oklahoma, purchased a copy of my *Heinerman's Encyclopedia of Healing Juices* (Englewood Cliffs, NJ: Prentice Hall, 1994). In thumbing through its pages, she found the "perfect cure" (as she called it) to her family's long history of allergies. Herewith are portions of her seven-page letter excerpted with her kind permission.

> "I purchased your book . . . early in '95. I was very interested in the experience you had with parsley and allergies. (See pages 186–189 of my *Encyclopedia of Healing Juices.*) My oldest daughter Cortne (16 at the time) was having serious trouble with allergies.

> "We were taking her to our family doctor for shots and other medications once a month or so . . . . It was all very expensive to say the least . . . . In the meantime our 12-year-old daughter, Eluce, was

working on a project for a science fair in school. She was also suffering from allergies. Our doctor said Tavist-D would be fine for her to take. It controlled her allergies, but made her dizzy and shakey [sic], even [with] $1/2$ then $1/4$ of the normal dosage.

"She decided to try the parsley recommended in your book for her allergies, and [for] her science fair project [too]. She began by drinking 4 T[ablespoons] of parsley juice in a small glass of carrot juice every morning. She had been congested upon [a]rising in the mornings. After 3–4 days this went away. It was working, but she hated the [taste of the] juice. A little pineapple juice added to the carrot juice seemed to improve the flavor for her.

"She kept track of the progress she was making in bringing her allergy symptoms under control. She did this for three weeks for her [school] project. While others in the family were [still] fighting allergies, she remained symptom-free. She made a nice display, and got a lot of interest at the science [sic] fair. Unfortunately, she stated her hypothesis wrong of why she thought the juice worked and only got 5th place. But she was still happy that her allergy no longer bothered her.

"After a week or so, [other] family members began to take notice. First, my husband gave it a try. The parsley juice worked well for him. But he preferred mixing it in with some V-8 juice instead on account of the taste. Then my 16-year-old gave it a try; she didn't seem to mind the taste at all. She took it straight—brave girl she was [for doing that]! By the end of the week we cancelled her appointment at the allergy clinic.

"She was in the middle of high school chemistry. They were studying the effects of prescription drugs on the body. A natural approach was starting to sound pretty good and she had seen results first hand. She still takes some Tavist-D occasionally. But most of the time the parsley juice controls it. She takes up to six T[ablespoons] of the juice a day, sometimes mixing it with a little apple, carrot, or tomato juice if she feels like it.

"Our son, 14, uses parsley only. His allergies aren't as bad, but he still suffers, and it is a source of relief for him as well. My husband usually would get two or three shots a year from our Dr., but this year he hasn't had one. Parsley juice is a quick, easy, effective alternative that takes effect in about 20 minutes. Thank you for sharing this simple but wonderful cure with America! God bless you in your research and writing efforts!"

Anthropological Research Center, which I've been the director of for the past 23 years, receives testimonials like this all the time. They are all very exciting to read, because they reconfirm the irrefutable fact that FOOD IS *ALWAYS* YOUR VERY *BEST* MEDICINE to take when you're not feeling so good!

Blood Poisoning Case Cured

Regarding one of the most unusual applications for parsley juice was described in a letter I received sometime ago from a toxicologist in Montgomery, Alabama, who shared with me his own experience with parsley juice.

> "I was bitten on the leg by what later turned out to be a brown recluse spider. As you probably know, such an arachnid bite can be quite lethal. I was hospitalized for five days and pumped full of antibiotics, but they only made me sicker. My leg swelled up and the area around the bite started festering and becoming gangrenous. Over the protests of my doctor, I forcibly checked myself out of the hospital and, with the assistance of family members, went back home.
>
> "My wife's aunt, who is well into her eighties, came by that night and brought some home remedies with her. Among them was a small pint jar of parsley juice. Using cotton balls and swabs dipped into some of the green juice, she cleaned the infected area around the bite. She applied a cotton pad soaked in the juice and taped it on the leg.
>
> "She also made me a drink of this juice. I swear I never tasted anything so gosh-awful in all my life. Though I'm not a drinker, I insisted that some scotch be added to not make it taste so horrible. Very reluctantly my wife added a little to each cup of parsley juice that I was forced to get down without gagging.
>
> "My aunt kept coming by every day to change the pad with a new one and make sure I was taking her juice. Within a week after this treatment started, the swelling and discoloration in my leg had nearly disappeared. I felt a lot better as a result of what my aunt did for me. She claimed that the parsley juice neutralized the poison in my body. Maybe it did and maybe it didn't; but I know one thing, for sure, that parsley juice probably saved my life!"

Woman's Anemia Corrected

Women always seem to need more iron than men do. A 27-year-old woman was suffering from fatigue. Her doctor told her she needed more iron. But instead of taking the iron tablets he prescribed, she decided to follow my suggestion of drinking a glass of carrot juice every day with $^1/_4$ cup of parsley juice mixed in with it. In 11 days her anemia situation was corrected and she had more energy after that.

PARSLEY JUICE SUPREME

Here's a simple way to make parsley juice. However, because of its rather zesty taste, you may want to dilute its invigorating flavor with a little apple, carrot, pineapple, or tomato juice.

> *1 bunch parsley, washed*
>
> *$^1/_2$ cup ice cubes*
>
> *$^1/_2$ cup mineral or spring water
>   (don't use tap water)*

Combine everything in a Vita-Mix whole food machine or similar food processor. Put the lid on the container and turn to the HIGH position. Blend for $1^1/_2$ minutes. Refrigerate. Use $^1/_3$ parsley juice with $^1/_3$ of any of the aforementioned juices three times a day or take it straight for control of allergy symptoms. And remember to *stay away from sugar and sugary foods!*

ALZHEIMER'S DISEASE

Utah Senior Regains Partial Memory with Bilberry Tea Extract

DESCRIPTION

Bilberry grows in the wild rather abundantly, being frequently found on shrub-covered hillsides or in heavily forested mountainous regions. It is a small shrub with wiry, angular branches that seldom exceed a foot in height. The flowers are globular in shape and waxy. The berries are jet black, but when overly ripe are covered with a delicate gray bloom.

The leaves of the bilberry shrub resemble those of the myrtle, being somewhat leathery. In the beginning they are rose-red, then yellowish-green, and they finally turn a fire-red in the fall. Their brilliant colors make them a decorative ornamental.

Partial Restoration of Memory with Tea

Alzheimer's disease is a health nightmare for older people; it is estimated to affect about 8 percent of those over age 65, about 12 percent of those between 75 and 85, and as many as 20 percent of those over 85.

This health problem results from the gradual degeneration of crucial neurons in the part of the brain that handles cognitive functioning. The onset of symptoms is often very slow. As symptoms progress, they tend to follow what doctors claim is an irreversible course. They begin with minor forgetfulness that becomes more pronounced over time and that culminates in profound loss of memory, identity, intellectual faculties, and control over bodily functions. In the final stages, severe mental impairment leads to complete dependence upon caregivers.

One woman who defied medical logic not long ago and actually reversed part of her *minor* memory loss is a 67 year old named Edith W. I became interested in her case because of something her daughter told me at a health convention at which I was speaking. This family member reported, "My mom has been drinking a tea that has reversed her memory loss."

When you hear a statement like that from someone in the middle of a crowd of people around you, it quickly grabs your attention—

at least it did mine. I virtually ignored everyone else around us clamoring for book autographs or answers to personal health questions and immediately focused on what this particular woman had to say. I took her off to the side, not far from the Author's Exhibit table, and queried her more carefully with regard to her remark.

She told me the following incredible story and I hastily scribbled shorthand notes of the same on a little pocket-size notebook I always carry with me for such interview purposes. Her name was Anne and she told me that her mom started experiencing memory lapses about two years before the time of our visit together (mid-1995).

Fearful that she would eventually become a "mindless zombie" (as she put it to her daughter), Edith began investigating whatever options were open for her. She read somewhere that Superoxide Dismutase (SOD)—an enteric coated enzyme supplement—and Coenzyme Q_{10} were good for this disease. She took 2 pills of SOD and 100 mg. of the other product each day with some of her meals. She did this for a while and noticed *some* improvement, but not the results she had expected to see.

A naturopathic doctor to whom she went for a medical consultation advised her to take a bilberry tea extract four times a day. She began doing this, and within weeks, her daughter claimed, she could begin to see a definite improvement in her mental capabilities. "Mom's mind just seemed to get sharper than it was before," Anne said with confidence. "Since doing the bilberry thing, she also has added Kyolic Garlic (4 capsules daily) and Ginkolic (2 capsules a day), both made by Wakunaga of America." To this I added $1/2$ glass of Pines' barley juice extract each day. "Just have your mom add 1 level teaspoonful of the Pines' barley juice extract powder in half a glass of water or vegetable juice, stir, and drink with a meal. Barley grass juice is one of the highest things in SOD," I concluded. (See Appendix for information on getting any of these fine products.)

I believe that the way that bilberry improves memory loss is by strengthening the tiny capillaries covering the entire brain, thereby promoting better blood circulation. A couple of capsules of cayenne pepper daily with food will nicely augment the bilberry tea for purposes of senile dementia and Alzheimer's.

Terrific Tea for Vision Improvement

Behind our eyes lies an elaborate network of very fine blood vessels. Any impairment in the circulation to them can decrease the delivery of important nutrients. This could eventually lead to vision problems such as cataracts, glaucoma, macular degeneration, and diabetic retinopathy. But European research has shown that bilberry extract protects the eyes from such diseases.

Italian researchers have reported that bilberry extract produces an 80 percent increase in blood circulation to the eyes and 80 percent improvement in vision. Keep in mind, though, that the extract is taken orally and *never* dropped into the eyes themselves. German doctors state that vitamin E oil (600 mg. daily) stopped the progression of cataract formation in 97 percent of their subjects tested. And a study published in a French medical journal showed that there was "significant improvement with bilberry" in 72 percent of people tested with nearsightedness, or myopia.

BILBERRY TEA EXTRACT

Go to a health food store or herb shop or order by mail from an herb supply house, some *whole* dried bilberries (you don't want the powder for making tea). In one pint of boiling water, put $1\frac{1}{4}$ tablespoons bilberries. Reduce heat, cover with lid, and simmer for 7 minutes. Set aside and steep another 40 minutes. Strain and refrigerate. Drink one *teacup* (or one-half regular cup) *warm* bilberry tea 4 times daily between meals.

BILBERRY FLUID EXTRACT

Combine 4 level tablespoons powdered bilberries with $1\frac{1}{2}$ cups good alcohol (Russian vodka or brandy are the best for this). You may dilute with $\frac{1}{3}$ cup distilled water if you wish. Let stand in jar for 2 weeks; shake often, then strain and store in another bottle. Take 15 drops under the tongue or in a little water three times a day.

AMENORRHEA

How Cheryl Started Her Monthly Periods Again with a Dynamic Vegetable Duo

DESCRIPTION

Carrot is high in certain important nutrients. Besides the well-known vitamin A, which definitely improves vision, this orange vegetable taproot is rich in potassium. Celery, on the other hand, with its green, fleshy petioles, is quite high in natural sodium content.

Apples always combine well with carrots and celery when they are being juiced together. Apples are rich in malic acid. The chemical interaction between both mineral salts and malic acid promotes the onset of normal menstruation.

Cheryl of Cincinnati Is Back in Business

Occasionally I get some of my juicing success stories from the strangest places. This one came from a woman in Cincinnati, Ohio, who asked that I use only her first name. Cheryl runs an escort service. But before your eyebrows rise and your stomach commences churning, let me hastily add (as she did) that is isn't *that* kind of escort service. "Our purpose is to provide accompaniment to senior citizens when they need to go to the supermarket, drugstore, post office, doctor's office, or bank," she said. "We most certainly are *not* in the business of providing voluptuous beauties to men of the 'lonely hearts club' who may be in need of a little female companionship!"

A while back Cheryl started noticing some physical signs indicative of amenorrhea. There was an absence of her monthly periods. A small milky discharge from both breast nipples became evident. Her body began manifesting a temperature intolerance. And she began experiencing unexplained food cravings and slight morning sickness even though she was definitely *not* pregnant. A visit to her doctor confirmed what she already suspected.

Cheryl decided to quit her escort business and devote her full time and attention to correcting this health problem before it became more serious. She had read in my other book *Encyclopedia of Healing Juices* (Englewood Cliffs, NJ: Prentice Hall, 1994) the back-to-back comments I had to say about carrot and celery juices (pp. 68–77).

Although I said nothing about either vegetable being good for amenorrhea, she figured that they might be of some assistance to her. "At the time I read your book," she told me by telephone, "I wasn't expecting them to do anything specific for my problem. But I though they could, at least, help me nutritionally."

Because she likes apples a lot, my informant decided to go ahead and add some to her vegetable drink mixture. "I was quite pleased to see just how well a little of this fruit improved the flavor of the carrots and celery," she remarked.

Cheryl drank one 8-ounce glass of this concoction in the morning and another glass at night. Within three days, she noted, "My menses were flowing again, and I was back to business as usual, thanks to these juices.

Juice Power 2 for the Ladies

6 baby carrots or $^1/_2$ cup carrots

$^1/_2$ cup celery

$^1/_2$ cup apple juice, bottled or canned

$^1/_2$ cup apples, preferably Granny Smith (green)

$^1/_4$ tsp. cinnamon powder

1 cup ice cubes

Place all the ingredients in their listed order in a Vita-Mix Total Nutrition Center or equivalent food blender. Make sure the lid is tightly secured beneath both tabs. Run the machine for $1^1/_2$ minutes until everything is smoothly mixed. Makes between 2 and 3 cups. Refrigerate. Divide in equal amounts for morning and evening consumption. It will be necessary to stir or briefly remix whatever remains in the refrigerator, as the microparticles of fiber pulp tend to settle.

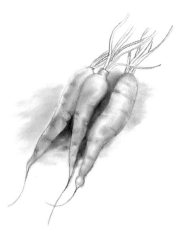

ANEMIA

Chlorophyll, the Key to Healthy Blood and Boundless Energy

DESCRIPTION

A more thorough description of the green pigment in plants has been given under AGING. Suffice it to say that "chlorophyll is to plant systems what blood is to human and animal bodies." Chlorophyll is remarkably high in organic iron, which is the crucial nutrient for those suffering from anemia. Women tend to suffer from *mild* anemia more than men do, and therefore require greater amounts of iron in their bodies.

Correcting Anemia and Giving Yourself More Energy

During the last quarter century, I have probably interviewed close to 600 or so folk healers and health-care providers worldwide. Many have been relatively uneducated by modern scientific standards, but have acquired vast empirical wisdom of considerable worth from their many years of folk healing experiences, which they have generously shared with me. A small percentage have been college trained and bring a different kind of knowledge to the health-care process.

The condition of anemia has been a fairly common one to treat for a large majority of these informants. In doing so, they each have obviously taken a number of different approaches. But a common thread among the many varied things they've recommended has been that which is *green.* In other words, sources of chlorophyll have been one of the principal agents routinely prescribed for general anemia. I've seen its success on numerous occasions and believe, with all my heart, that *it is the key* to correcting the several different types of this blood disorder.

One of my favorite chlorophyll drinks for giving the blood system a great nutritional boost is actually an adaptation of several vegetable drink recipes developed by Rose Wride and her staff at the Vita-Mix Test Kitchen in Cleveland, Ohio, and which is included in their *Total Nutrition Center Recipe and Instruction Book* (Cleveland: Vita-Mix Corp., 1993; p. 159).

I've recommended this version of my Green Drink to many of those who've been bothered with one form or another of anemia at some time in their lives. About 85 percent of those who've gone to the effort to make the drink for themselves using a Vita-Mix Whole Food Machine (or equivalent blender) have reported feeling stronger and more mentally alert and having increased appetite, modest weight gain, better skin appearance, normal heart rhythm, and, in a few instances, even darker hair color. These changes come about slowly and take several months to be eventually realized.

IRON-FORTIFIED GREEN DRINK FOR BOUNDLESS ENERGY

This is one of my favorite chlorophyll recipes. It is an amalgam of several different juice recipes borrowed from the recipe book published by the Vita-Mix Corp. and used here with their kind permission.

> *1 cup pineapple juice, chilled*
>
> *1 cup papaya juice, chilled (dilute from concentrate, if necessary)*
>
> *1 tsp. each lime and lemon juices*
>
> *$1/_4$ cup celery stalk, chopped, with leaves intact*
>
> *$1/_4$ cup spinach leaves*
>
> *$1/_4$ cup parsley sprigs*
>
> *$1/_4$ cup peppermint leaves, cut*
>
> *$1/_4$ cup spring water*
>
> *1 cup ice cubes*

Place all the ingredients in the Vita-Mix container in the order given. Secure the complete two-part lid by locking it under the tabs. Move the black speed control level to HIGH. Then lift the black lever to the ON position and allow the machine to run for almost 2 minutes, until everything is of a smooth consistency. Makes approximately 2 cups.

And where it isn't always convenient to make up this green drink due to lack of time or kitchen facilities, there are alternatives available. They come in the form of *dried* chlorophyll powders. One of the most common brands on the market at present is Pines Wheat Grass by Pines International. I generally recommend mixing one tablespoon of the Pines Wheat Grass in an 8-fluid-ounce glass of spring or mineral water or tomato or carrot juice. It is good to stir in one tablespoon of Pines Organic Beet Juice Powder. This will give additional iron from another vegetable source, which people with anemia (especially women) need very much. (See Product Appendix for more information.)

Along with this I always recommend that 2 to 3 tablets of a high-potency B-complex vitamin supplement be taken. Another thought is to add a teaspoon of desiccated liver powder to such an instant chlorophyll drink. Some even stir in a little brewer's yeast and blackstrap molasses. With all these things in place, the problem of anemia should be corrected in no time at all.

ANGER

FedEx Driver Calmed with Chamomile Tea After Theft of Machine Gun

DESCRIPTION

There are two different species of chamomile. German chamomile is an annual herb growing up to 20 inches. It has an erect, much branched, cylindrical stem and light-green leaves that are finely divided and almost feathery-looking. Single daisylike flowerheads, an inch wide, grow on long stalks and have yellow centers and white petal-like ray flowers. The blooms have an applelike smell to them. This is the type of chamomile that is very popular in Austria, Hungary, Germany, Belgium, Luxembourg, and Switzerland. It is the better selling of the two chamomiles in the American health food and herb industries.

Roman chamomile, on the other hand, is more popular in Wales, Scotland, Ireland, and Great Britain. As readers of *The Tale of Peter Rabbit* may recall from their childhood, it was this kind of chamomile that Peter's mother gave to him after he had overindulged in Mr. McGregor's vegetable garden. It closely resembles German chamomile, both having pale-green, feathery-looking leaves, both producing daisylike flowers, and both emitting an unmistakable applelike fragrance.

A Rousing Tale of Anger Calmed with Tea

It is not very often that I get an herbal healing story involving the use of firearms, particularly a narrative featuring the kind of weapon that the fictional British spy James Bond (Agent 007 in the books and movies) might sometimes resort to.

Well, such a high-tech machine was actually stolen from a delivery truck during the third week of July 1995 after federal agents in the Beehive State of Utah sent it to San Francisco, California, via Federal Express. The Utah-built weapon was a .22-caliber machine gun mounted inside an ordinary briefcase that any business person might use. The gun could be fired by pressing a button on the briefcase handle. The weapon was aimed by activating a laser sight that put a red dot of light on the target, according to several Bureau of Alcohol,

Tobacco and Firearms (ATF) agents with whom I spoke by phone concerning this matter.

This novel briefcase weapon was confiscated a decade ago in a raid by federal law enforcement officers on a Utah gun-manufacturing business. The fancy weapon was part of a routine shipment of guns from one ATF office to another. The machine gun that would delight the mythical British secret agent 007 was in one of three boxes shipped from my state. The boxes contained a total of 18 weapons, including shotguns, handguns, and other machine guns.

All the weapons being shipped had been previously confiscated in connection with criminal investigations. ATF had the option of destroying such weapons or keeping them for educational purposes. Since all of them, including the briefcase special, were fully operational, the decision was made to save them for training new agents.

But something quite unexpected happened in San Francisco. A Federal Express truck driver was followed by several enterprising thieves as he made deliveries along his route. While he carried a small package inside a building at one stop, the thieves quickly hit his truck, making off with six boxes of computer equipment—and a seventh box of approximately the same dimensions containing the James Bond-type weapon.

I spoke by telephone with the unnamed driver at his home in Foster City (just below San Francisco) several weeks later, after learning about the incident from employees in the Federal Express office in downtown Salt Lake City. The driver insisted that his identity remain anonymous before agreeing to speak with me. I guaranteed it would.

He figured that "these crooks were probably following me for the computers I was carrying, and not for any of the AFT property I had in the truck with me." The driver said the whole ordeal "upset me very much, made me mad as hell." He said after reporting the incident to his supervisors and answering numerous questions from the police and ATF agents, "I went home in one of the worst moods I believe I've ever been in in my life."

But the driver's wife, who happened to be "a health food nut" (as he humorously described her to me), brewed up some chamomile tea for him to drink. She boiled a pint of water and put into it six chamomile tea bags, "probably more than she usually does," he assumed, "because my feelings were pretty intense that evening." She covered the teapot with its lid and let the tea bags steep for 30 minutes before pouring her husband a cup of warm tea. She sweetened it with a little honey and added "a touch" of pure vanilla extract to "help flavor it more for me," he said.

"As I started sipping that warm, delicious brew," he continued, "I was amazed at how gently it started working on my nervous system. Within minutes I felt more relaxed than I had been all day long. Not only did the tension in my muscles seem to melt away, but the stress built up inside of me also appeared to be waning. I don't know how to explain it to you any better than this, Dr. Heinerman. But it was like all of my anger at the thieves and disgust I felt toward myself for not being more attentive just seemed to evaporate into thin air.

"I don't know what it was in the tea that did it," he concluded, "but it sure worked wonders for me." He questioned if "maybe the temperature of the tea may have had something to do with how I felt." I said it was probably that, the tea itself, as well as the vanilla his wife added for flavoring.

I've tried the chamomile tea since then when I've been a little upset with something and discovered that it didn't work as well alone as it did when $1/2$ teaspoon of pure vanilla extract was added to it while the tea was still *hot*.

Terrific for Colds and Influenza

An old European naturopathic doctor once told me years ago that drinking "several cups of hot chamomile tea, laced with rum or brandy, if possible, will bring on a good sweat" in someone who has a bad cold or a nasty case of the flu. He raved about what a "great sweat-inducing agent" this herb was, which prompted me to jokingly dub chamomile "a terrific sudorific!"

He always made the tea in large quantities, so it could be drunk copiously like water by his sick patients. Usually a quart or more of water was boiled before two cups of chamomile flowers were added. They were stirred with a spoon, covered with a lid, and allowed to steep for nearly an hour. A glass of tea would then be strained, slightly reheated, and given to the patient to drink. The treatment would be repeated every hour. At the same time the sick person would be stripped naked and wrapped in an old white sheet and several heavy wool blankets. This would induce a mighty sweat that would release from the body considerable poisons.

Everyone on whom he used this treatment always recovered very quickly from their colds or flus. He was of the definite opinion that "a strong, hot cup of chamomile tea will greatly benefit someone who is sick with respiratory disorders like these."

Soothes Stomach Problems

My grandmother on my father's side, Barbara Leibhardt Heinerman, was a folk healer from the old country of Temesvara, Hungary (now part of Romania). She knew a lot about herbs and doctored not only my dad, Jacob Heinerman, when he was a kid, but also both of her grandsons, namely my brother Joseph and me when we were very young and occasionally not feeling well.

She had a stomach complaint for many years that didn't permit her a wide variety of food. Her diet was very limited in the things she could eat. Chicken soup with crackers, a little cooked cereal, some plain baked bread, a little homemade yogurt or cottage cheese, and so forth, was the best she could manage.

But to help control her problem and relieve most of the gastrointestinal discomforts she might otherwise have suffered, she resorted to drinking warm chamomile tea several times a day. When I was old enough to understand such things, my father told me how much it helped for this as well as for soothing her jumpy nerves.

One of my other health reference books, *Heinerman's Encyclopedia of Healing Herbs and Spices* (Englewood Cliffs, NJ: Prentice Hall, 1995) has more information in it on this wonderful herbal tea and tonic. Readers interested in learning more of its uses are encouraged to consult that book.

MAKING A WONDERFUL CUP OF CHAMOMILE

My dad's mother, God rest her soul, brewed a great cup of chamomile that even a fussy five year old like myself at the time enjoyed savoring the aroma and sipping the delicious flavor. Here's how Grandmother Barbara did it:

> *1 pint boiling water*
>
> *$2^1/_4$ tsps. dried cut chamomile flowers*
>
> *tiny dash pure vanilla flavoring*

Put the herbal flowers in the boiling water; cover with lid, set aside, and let steep for 10 minutes. Uncover and add the vanilla. Then re-cover and steep some more for an additional 10 minutes. Strain and drink *warm*. The dash of vanilla really gives it an unbeatable flavor.

ANGINA

A Tonifying Tea Formula for a Common Heart-Lung-Blood Disorder

DESCRIPTION

There are essentially three main herbs that make up a very special tea I formulated years ago. They are hawthorn berries, ginger root, and peppermint leaves.

The hawthorn can be either a deciduous shrub or a tree with stout branches, growing up to 40 feet in height. The smooth leaves have 3 to 7 lobes. The attractive white or pink flowers are followed by oval red fruits that contain one seed apiece.

Ginger root has been common in the ancient medical systems of India and Greece for many, many centuries. It was eventually acquired by Europeans from Arab merchants through trade and barter. Today the best ginger comes from Jamaica. The gnarled and knobby rhizome is encased in a delicate, silvery-brown skin; when made into a tea, it imparts a warm, pungent tang.

Peppermint is a perennial herb and shares square stems and the method of spreading by means of runners with spearmint and penny-royal. Peppermint is 3 feet tall, has toothed, oblong-to-oval, stalked leaves up to 2 inches in length. The lilac-pink flowers grow in dense, club-shaped spikes. More than any other plant that I know of, peppermint is probably one of the best herbs for getting more oxygen into the body. And while herbalists may extol its virtues in *fresh* form, I like to sing its praises when it is utilized dried.

Some Helpful Tips for Dealing with Angina

Angina is a very serious medical condition. It requires prompt attention by a doctor as soon as possible. In a high number of angina cases, impending heart attacks aren't too far behind. A doctor can diagnose angina on the basis of elicited symptoms. Medical tests such as an exercise stress test or coronary angiography (a special X-ray study of the heart's circulation) are at a doctor's disposal to better evaluate angina.

Believe it or not, something as life threatening as this can be easily controlled by making a few necessary lifestyle changes. These will help to lower the heart's workload and reduce stress. A good night's sleep and afternoon cat naps help a lot. So do morning and evening walks or leisure strolls. Some *slow* stretching exercises, such as those advocated in hatha yoga or tai-ji-quan are also quite useful.

The heart's demand for oxygen may also be modified with natural substances. A winning formula I developed years ago and have been successfully recommending for several hundred angina cases ever since calls for hawthorn berries, peppermint leaves, and ginger root. It is something I came up with after watching folk healers in other cultures use different herbs to treat their angina patients. I adopted the three best into my own combination. The formula is given at the end of this section.

Other things can be done to decrease the risk of an angina attack. You need first to identify and then control those factors that contribute to chest pain. For instance, avoid running up a flight of stairs or racing to catch a bus or being outdoors on cold, windy days. Take your time and *never* hurry; it isn't worth it in terms of what can happen to your health. Use common sense and dress warmly in inclement weather. Don't leave anything to chance. Anger and stress can provoke angina, so be at peace with yourself in mind and heart.

If you happen to be one of those proverbial "couch potatoes" we hear so much about these days, I highly recommend a medically supervised exercise-conditioning program that will help increase your tolerance to physical activity. The right kind of exercise can also improve your heart function and assist in building collateral circulation to the heart muscle.

Angina tends to be a progressive disorder and is commonly (but not always) a predictor of a heart attack. With some individuals the condition may continue for many years with little change. Others, though, might experience the increasingly frequent or severe attacks of unstable angina. The pain of angina in and of itself isn't dangerous, but it's a definite clarion call to potential heart disease.

Those who smoke should stop! And those who are exposed to second-hand smoke should change their breathing environment if at all possible. Obese people should change their diet, eat several light meals a day rather than fewer larger ones, rest after eating, and engage in moderate exercise of some kind. Avoid cold weather and reduce tension around you.

Angina Tea Reduces Hypertension

Over the years, I've heard from a number of those who've been greatly helped by my angina tea formula. One of the more common problems that it seems nicely to have alleviated is high blood pressure. People report that after they start drinking some of the tea on a regular basis their blood pressure slowly goes down to within a more normal range.

Helps Asthma and Bronchitis

A few of those who've been bothered with respiratory disorders claimed it was my tea combination that helped them breathe better again. They always took it *very warm,* one cup at a time, and usually between meals. They've also reported that taking it an hour before bedtime enabled them to breathe better while resting in bed.

JOHN'S ANTI-ANGINA TEA

1²/₃ quarts boiling water

³/₄ cup hawthorn berries

¹/₄ cup grated ginger root

1 cup peppermint leaves

1 tsp. pure vanilla extract

1 tsp. blackstrap molasses

Boil the water first. Then add the hawthorn berries and ginger root. Cover and reduce heat, simmering for 10 minutes. Then set aside, uncover, and add the peppermint leaves. Stir thoroughly, cover again, and let steep for 15 minutes. Uncover and add the last two ingredients. Cover again and continue steeping for an additional 25 minutes. Strain and refrigerate. Reheat one cup amounts and drink on an empty stomach several times a day.

ANOREXIA

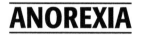

(see Anxiety, Bulimia, and Underweight)

ANXIETY

Hysterical Woman Put at Ease with Valerian-Skullcap Potion

DESCRIPTION

Valerian is a perennial herb that grows up to 5 feet in height. The stem is erect. Opposite leaves are divided into 5 to 12 pairs of leaflets, which become smaller, narrower, and feathery toward the top of the stem. Tiny, sweet-scented, white-to-pale-pink flowers grow in long-stalked clusters at the end of the stem. The root is the medicinal part and emits a smell of sweaty socks or stinky shorts when it starts to dry.

Skullcap is another perennial herb, but with an erect, smooth, branching stem growing only to a yard at the most. Broadly lance-shaped, toothed leaves grow in opposite pairs. Small tubular blue, pinkish, violet, or white flowers have two lips, the upper one hooded.

Plumb Scared out of Her Wits, but Calmed Down with an Herbal Tea

What I'm about to relate is, as they swear in a court of law, "the truth, the whole truth, and nothing but the truth, so help me God." The reason I preface it this way, is because the accounts I'm about to relate are two of the most unusual I've ever heard about. Besides being scary, however, they are also very funny at the end.

The tales come from a Mormon family history book entitled *Letters to Mary (1879–1929)* by Helen Bay Gibbons (Salt Lake City: Helen Bay Gibbons, Publisher, 1972, pp. 65–66). The contents consist of hundreds of letters written to a devout woman, Mary Eva Bay, who passed away in her nineties many years ago. The following narrative excerpts pick up sometime in the last quarter century of the 1800s and took place in one of the small communities located in South-central Utah. Probably more than anything else I've come across, they typify what true anxiety can be about, though in a most extraordinary way.

> "Sickness in a small isolated community, without doctors, druggists, or morticians could be a very serious matter. The people usually had to rely upon themselves in caring for the sick or

dying. Home remedies were tried, with herbs gathered by certain local herb 'experts' often being called upon. Only in extreme circumstances would the doctor . . . be called. It meant two round trips of about a hundred miles by horseback or buggy—one for the person sent to get the doctor and the other to take him back. And then, often by the time he could get the word and get [there] it was too late anyway.

"In the event of a death, women of the town [of Junction, Utah] would help each other to wash, clothe, and prepare the body for burial, while the men would build the coffin, dig the grave, and lower the body into the ground themselves. Having no embalming fluid or mortuary service, burial would take place as soon as possible after death. While waiting for the funeral—usually the following day, the body would be packed in ice, and women of the town would take turns 'sitting up with the dead' to change the ice packs and keep the corpse chilled all through the night.

"To women inexperienced in this kind of gruesome assignment, it was a fearful duty. On one occasion, a woman friend of the deceased was called to the home soon after death to care for the corpse. Weeping as she washed her dead friend's arm, she raised it only to have the fingers close, as if clutching at her. Not realizing that this was a normal muscle reflex before the stiffness of rigor mortis set in, she was horrified. She ran from the room crying: 'We're burying Ivy alive! She's not dead yet!'

"The dead bodies would be placed in the coolest possible place for the night's vigil, and this sometimes meant the cellar of a home. One night, a rather nervous woman assigned to take the midnight to six A.M. shift, changing dressings and watching over the dead, posted herself in a room adjoining the cool room where the corpse lay.

"In the silence of the night, she began to hear unmistakable signs of labored breathing from the other room, as though someone were trying to clear fluids from their throat. It was a kind of gurgling sound. With a sense of horror, she carried the flickering lamp into the room to investigate. Only the still, white form of the dead lay there upon the slab, cold and stiff.

"'Oh, it was my imagination!' she scolded herself and returned to the book she was reading in the other room.

"But as things grew quiet again, she heard the gurgling sound once more, only this time louder and more prolonged. Stifling a scream, she ran to the neighbors and awakened them, afraid to return alone to the makeshift morgue.

"When her companions returned with her to the cool room, they, like her, found the corpse unmoving, very definitely dead! But then, in the same room, they, too, heard the ominous gurgle, like labored breathing. Turning the light about, they finally saw on a shelf a bottle of home-preserved fruit which was spoiling. The fermentation periodically forced open the lid a crack, and when it bubbled over, the pressure released, was silent once again."

Needless to say, both women in each case, suffered "anxiety attacks" for the next several days. Mary, who heard of these things and knew each Mormon woman intimately, referred them to a local herb doctor living in the area. He went out into the nearby foothills, taking with him a small spade and an old gunny sack.

Soon he located some fragrant valerian growing wild. He knew it was valerian because of the unmistakable aroma emitted and the plant's distinctive small, reddish flowers. Once he had excavated some roots and quickly sniffed them, he knew from the "dirty socks" smell that they were what he was after.

He walked a short distance to another spot, where a yard-tall perennial with two-lipped blue flowers was gently swaying in the breeze. This was the skullcap he needed, and he chopped it off at its base with the point of his shovel. He stuffed the whole plant inside the sack and returned to his home in Junction an hour later.

Although his name was never given in the reference previously cited, details about his method of preparation were, fortunately enough, provided. He washed the valerian roots in some cold water and then sliced them lengthwise before cutting each one in half-inch diagonal circles. What must have amounted to about $2^1/_2$ to $3^1/_4$ cups of valerian roots was then tossed into a black iron kettle of boiling water (estimated to have been equal to two quarts of fluid). Here they cooked uncovered for roughly 30 minutes. Then several handfuls (maybe two or three) of coarsely chopped skullcap plant were added, and a heavy lid put over the top. The kettle was then pushed to one side and toward the back of the coal-wood stove, where the contents could simmer without further heavy cooking.

About two hours afterward he strained this brew through some clean muslin and discarded the herb materials. He now had a pretty strong tea. He filled two quart bottles with it and eventually gave one to each of the women who had been adversely affected during their separate periods of "death watch." He instructed each of them to take what amounted to 3 cups at one time of his brew twice a day, if need be. Such a large dose or draft of liquid medicine was in former times called a potion.

It was reliably reported that within 48 hours each woman had overcome her "anxiety attacks" and no longer felt threatened by things either real or imagined.

Paranoia Overcome

A while back I happened to be visiting with a friend of mine who is a mental health care provider in a local psychiatric hospital. Since he is a history buff just as I am, I read to him both accounts from *Letters to Mary.* It really cracked him up to hear the reactions of each woman in her particular and unusual situation. I also briefly informed him what the town herbalist did for them.

At this point in our conversation, the humor ceased and he became very focused on the remedy part of both stories. He asked me very seriously if such a thing today might help someone troubled with paranoia. He said he had a sister who suffered from this period- ic derangement. He claimed she demonstrated systematized delu- sions, though often of a persecutory character, in an otherwise intact personality.

I told him that he, not I, was the mental health expert here. But, I noted, "It wouldn't hurt to give it a try." I had him reduce the water and herbs by half and purchase both botanicals, already packaged, from a local health food store in the city. He discovered he had to sweeten the tea with some sugar before his sister agreed to take it. Later on, when we got together again and I inquired of her progress, he said that daily use of that potion had greatly reduced her symp- toms and made her "fairly normal" again.

AN ANTI-ANXIETY TEA THAT'S PALATABLE

Anyone who had ever had the unhappy misfortune of tasting valerian root *tea* will know that it is one of those strongly medicinal herbs with a yucky taste as well as an icky smell to it. But for treating anxiety, the root works best when made as a tea. So the challenge to me was to try and find a way to make something nasty tasting into more of a flavorful beverage.

Now that's a pretty tall order, I must admit, but I set out determined to come up with something better than what Nature herself had offered up. After a little bit of "trial-and-error" testing, here's what I finally came up with.

> *1 level tsp. of finely chopped or powdered dried valerian root*
>
> *1 tsp. cut, dried, or powdered dried skullcap plant*
>
> *$1/_4$ tsp. mace*

> $^1/_4$ **tsp. powdered cardamon**
>
> $^1/_4$ **tsp. dark honey**
>
> **1 pint boiling water**

Simmer the valerian root in the water, covered with a lid, on low heat for 5 minutes. Then add the skullcap and steep for 10 minutes. Uncover and add the two spices. Cover and steep again for another 10 minutes.

Then strain the contents through a fine wire-mesh strainer or layered cheesecloth and return to the pan. Gently reheat, uncovered, until quite warm. Then add the honey, stirring thoroughly until well blended with the tea. Refrigerate and drink one cup *cool* (but not cold), twice daily if needed.

ARTERIOSCLEROSIS/ ATHEROSCLEROSIS

A Great Juice Workout for the Cardiovascular System

DESCRIPTION

Garlic and onion are popular spices the world over. They add flavor and greatly improve the taste of whatever foods they're added to. The sulfur compounds contained in them help to lower serum cholesterol and triglyceride levels. By doing to they help to prevent hardening of the arteries.

Aged garlic extract from Japan is a unique herbal product. The Wakunaga Pharmaceutical Company of Hiroshima, together with a German scientist, developed and patented a process many years ago that took garlic from the field and subjected it to a lengthy period of fermentation. During this time a number of important things happen. For one, the offensive odor virtually disappears. For another, the vitamin and mineral content of many vital nutrients increases. Enzyme activity also notably increases as well. Finally, some of the negative reactions that a portion of the population might be apt to experience are done away with. A case in point is the strong hypoglycemic activity present in *raw* garlic. For diabetics this is good, but for people already suffering from low blood sugar this comes as bad news since it can aggravate existing symptoms. However, when garlic is subjected to several months of intense "aging" this allergic side effect disappears. Japanese aged garlic extract is sold throughout the world under the brand name Kyolic; it is considered by many doctors and scientists to be *the* world's premier selling commercial garlic product. It is widely available in health food stores and nutrition centers.

Parsley and celery are quite high in calcium, magnesium, phosphorus, potassium, and iron, not to mention vitamins A and C. Their mineral-rich composition helps to prevent cholesterol buildup on the artery walls of the heart. They do this by making individual red blood cells less sticky and by assisting the colon in eliminating greater amounts of excess cholesterol.

Cayenne pepper and ginger root are two spices known to increase the circulation of blood throughout the body. Quite often the blood platelets can become sticky; when this happens they tend to bunch up like grapes. Such clustering effects can lead to blood clots and potential strokes. But cayenne and ginger, along with celery and parsley, are able to reduce this stickiness so that platelets can slide over each other better and move more freely through the system.

"Juice Workout" Saved This Man's Heart

Mark W. is a 53-year-old logger from the city of Coeur d'Alene, located in the top part of the Idaho panhandle. He started experiencing periodic chest pains, labored breathing, and abnormal conditions of the heart involving premature beats, irregular rhythms, rapid cardiac rate (about 100 beats per minute), slight murmur, and some enlargement.

He went to a cardiologist, who leaned toward alternative medicine somewhat and prescribed things beyond the scope of surgery and drugs. Mark was diagnosed as having atherosclerotic heart disease. Among the checklist of items prescribed to him by his doctor were these:

- Stop smoking.
- Stop breathing second-hand smoke.
- Increase daily exercise through moderate walking.
- Reduce fat intake by 70 percent.
- Cut sugar intake by 50 percent.
- Stop drinking coffee and colas.
- Eat more raw foods, including salads.
- Enroll in a medically supervised weight-loss program.
- Get blood cholesterol tested every 2 weeks.
- Get blood pressure tested monthly.
- Stop worrying and be happier.

Mark went on this program for one month and noticed some modest signs of improvement. He was able to breathe again without much difficulty. And the function of his heart had returned to a slightly better pace. But the chest pains still persisted, and a second diagnosis from the same doctor showed that nothing had been done to reduce his cardiomegaly, or swelling.

His wife contacted me by telephone and wanted to know what else could be done to help her husband get rid of his chest pains and the heart enlargement. I told her about a particular juice program that I had specifically developed a few years ago just for the cardiovascular system. I gave her the ingredients and simple instructions on how to make it over the phone and asked her to let me know in six weeks or so how he was doing.

A little more time than that passed before she called me again. By then nearly $2^1/_2$ months had elapsed. Because I frequently get many calls from people all over the country asking for folk wisdom advice relative to simple problems, I couldn't recall her name until she refreshed my memory with some brief facts about her husband's case. She then proceeded to tell me how much the juice formula had helped Mark. "Now my husband is able to go out and put in a full day logging without any pain or discomfort," she said. The woman attributed this good news to what the cardiologist had prescribed and to my "juice workout," as I call it. The recipe is found at the end of this section.

Assistance for Circulatory Disorders

Older people tend to experience more circulatory disorders than do younger individuals. Part of this may come from the inevitable process of aging. Other factors leading to coldness in the lower extremities, venous insufficiency, and varicose veins may be poor diet and lack of adequate exercise.

One-half glass of this juice every day with a meal will show improvement in the circulatory system. Blood flow will become pretty well normalized, and related disorders will be minimized. People who've given my "Juice Workout" a try have reported feeling stronger action in their cardiovascular systems. The ingredients really are good for the old ticker after all!

Juice Workout for the Old Ticker

Now for the part featuring my dynamic juice therapy. I am firmly committed to juices for improving a person's health, because they offer the body the equivalent of a good physical workout in a gym lifting and pressing weights. The juice program I'm about to recommend gives the cardiovascular system terrific exercise if faithfully consumed every day.

Juice Workout for the Old Ticker

1 cup canned tomato juice

$1/_2$ cup mineral tonic water

1 raw garlic clove, peeled

2 tbsp. liquid Kyolic garlic (see Product Appendix)

3 tbsp. raw onion (preferably sweet onion)

$1/_2$ bunch of parsley

$1/_2$ cup celery, with leaves

$1/_2$ vegetarian bouillon cube (extra large size)

1 tsp. granulated kelp

pinches of powdered cayenne pepper and ginger root

1 cup ice cubes

Put everything into a Vita-Mix Total Nutrition Center (or equivalent food machine), carefully secure the lid, and turn on to HIGH for 2 minutes. Drink at least 1 glass of this each day. And since cold liquids are apt to produce a slight shock to the body, it may be advisable to either drink this at *room temperature* or to eliminate the ice cubes and *not* refrigerate.

ARTHRITIS

Fifty-Eight-Year-Old Telephone Sales Rep Finds Relief with Apple-Mixed Greens Drink

DESCRIPTION

The common apple was once considered a species of the same genus that pears come from because of the same characteristic pome fruit that both share. Apples are native to the Caucasus mountains of Western Asia and have been under extensive cultivation for the last several thousand years.

The *Book of Mormon* (a record of ancient America) tells about a people called the Jaredites, who emigrated from the Tower of Babel somewhere in central Iraq to the Western Hemisphere around 2000 B.C. It tells of them brining along a wide variety of fruit and vegetable seeds, animals, fish in tanks, bees (called Deseret), and a lot of their own personal effects. It is believed by some scientists who specialize in plant genetics that some of the apples of Central and South America had their earliest origins from this part of Central Asia.

Parsley and spinach are rich in important mineral salts such as calcium, magnesium, potassium, phosphorous, and some sodium. When these alkaline trace elements are combined with the natural sugars and enzymes in apples, the inflammation accompanying joint tenderness and swelling often goes away.

Saleslady Becomes Pain-Free

One of the many joys derived from being a writer of successful health books is to either meet in person or speak with by telephone some of the countless people I've had a chance to influence for good in this life. Especially gratifying, however, is when someone tells me how he or she may have been helped by something recommended in one of my books.

On Thursday, October 5, 1995, I had the wonderful opportunity to chat with such an individual long distance. Her name is Carol Galippo and she was then 58 years old. She works as a telephone sales representative for a large manufacturer and distributor of fine consumer products in Cleveland, Ohio.

Toward the latter part of 1994, she began experiencing considerable lower back pain. "If I sat for long hours at a time without getting up and moving around," she began, "then I would be very stiff

40

and hurt all over." So she consulted with an orthopedic surgeon, who diagnosed her problem as degenerative arthritis of the spine.

"He prescribed for me a strong drug called Relafen," she continued. "I started taking two pills a day sometime in January [of 1995]. While it did help my back pain go away, it created another, equally severe problem. My stomach started hurting. Eventually the pain became so intense that I could hardly tolerate it. I went back to my doctor, who then readjusted the dosage to only one pill a day. But, while that stopped my stomach pains, it wasn't enough for my back, which started hurting all over again. I was at my wits' end as to what I should do.

"A copy of your *Encyclopedia of Healing Juices* (Englewood Cliffs, NJ: Prentice Hall, 1995) came to my attention. And I flipped through it to see what might be good for my problem. I read on page 8 of your book that *fermented* apple juice was good for arthritis. I also discovered elsewhere in the volume that parsley and spinach were very helpful for pain and inflammation.

"So I decided to give your recommendations a try. I thought to myself, 'What do I have to lose?' I know you praised the Granny Smith variety of apples, so I made sure to get them. I bought some bottled organic apple juice as well. I juiced one-half an apple with a small amount of the regular apple juice in the morning before going to work and let it stand at room 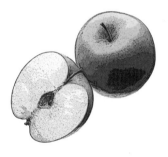 temperature until late in the evening. By then it usually had started to 'work' a little, indicating some fermentation was setting in. I also washed and got ready my parsley and spinach leaves and put them in the refrigerator until they were needed.

"Just before retiring, I made up my special juice and drank one glass of it always on an empty stomach before going to bed. I was amazed at how quickly this stuff worked. I mean, within days I could tell a difference. Most of the soreness and pain left me and I am now able to sit long hours in a chair at my work station, taking phone calls and giving out sales pitches without any more suffering.

"There are about five or six other ladies here in the company who also suffer from arthritis and I've been showing them your juice book and telling them just how fantastically this apple-mixed greens drink really works. You have no idea how many of us with this kind of back problem or other arthritic conditions you've been able to help."

Bye-Bye Pain Drink

For want of a better name, this is what I've elected to call my informant's novel concoction. She told me outright before I even had a chance to ask her "I juice everything with a Vita-Mix. I trust *no other* machine. I've been using a Vita-Mix for 20 years and I wouldn't trade it away for anything in the world." Then pausing for a brief moment, she added with a laugh, "except maybe for a newer model."

> $1/_2$ *Granny Smith apple*
>
> $1/_4$ *cup organic apple juice*
>
> $1/_2$ *bunch parsley, washed and refrigerated*
>
> *6–8 large fresh spinach leaves, washed and refrigerated*
>
> *OR*
>
> *8–10 small fresh spinach leaves, washed and refrigerated*
>
> $1/_2$ *cup ice cubes*

When inquiring about specific amounts for each ingredient, Ms. Galippo laughed over the telephone and remarked: "In all the years I've been cooking and following recipes, I don't believe I've ever gone by any exact amount. I do things by handfuls as a rule."

Prepare the apple and apple juice as previously described. But blend it for only 1 minute, then set aside in a warm part of your kitchen for about 10 to 12 hours for a slight fermentation to set in. Return it to the Vita-Mix machine and add the rest of the ingredients. Blend for 2 minutes. Drink just before retiring for the night.

Aztec Tonic Kept 99-Year-Old Hispanic Woman Arthritis-Free

There are several different types of arthritis: degenerative arthritis (also known as osteoarthritis); infectious arthritis; psoriatic arthritis (also called psoriasis); rheumatoid arthritis (RA); spinal arthritis (also called ankylosing spondylitis); and traumatic arthritis.

The most common of these is rheumatoid arthritis (hereafter cited as RA); it also happens to be one of the most severe forms of the disease as well. It is estimated that close to 11 million Americans are affected in some way by RA. It can begin at just about any age, but ordinarily strikes people in their thirties and forties and affects women three times more often than it does men.

The exact cause of RA remains a mystery to medical science; all that researchers know so far is that somehow the immune system is involved. Instead of protecting the body from disease, the immune system attacks the joints, causing inflammation that damages the joints. Heredity may play a role in some people; in others, a viral infection may trigger the process. Some doctors think that a substance they've named rheumatoid factor could also be involved in the disease process.

RA is a chronic disease that typically comes and goes, flaring up and then going into remissions that could last for weeks, months, or even years. It can be severely painful and can cause permanent damage to joints, as well as affecting other organs of the body. On the other hand, it could be mild and have little or no effect. Although RA is often painful and crippling, it isn't dangerous, as such.

The classic symptoms of RA include:

- swelling, pain, tenderness, or warmth in one or more joints, usually symmetrically in both sides of the body;
- joint stiffness, especially upon awakening in the morning;
- an inability to move a joint normally;
- unexplained weight loss, fever, or weakness;
- a general malaise.

The Solution

From 1993 to 1996 my family resided at 1071 South Blair Street in Salt Lake City. It is near historic Liberty Park, which is this city's answer to Manhattan's Central Park. Blair Street sits like the horizontal line in the capital letter *H*, with the two side streets of Herbert and Harvard Avenues, respectively, forming its left and right vertical lines.

Half a block north of us and just around the corner on Herbert Avenue lived an elderly Hispanic lady by the name of Augustine Ramona Atencio Gurule. Had her relatives listened to her tearful pleadings and *not* acted improperly by putting her into a rest home in Provo, but instead left her in her own house, she would certainly have reached age 100 by August 28, 1995. As it was, though, her tenacious will to live immediately ceased, and within a week of the unhappy transfer south, she had "given up the ghost" and vacated her mortal remains. Gone for good was this descendant of an ancient Aztec princess.

But while she was alive, she was the kind of good soul you might come to expect in an aged grandma. Her numerous descendants included many grandchildren, great-grandchildren, and great-great-grandchildren who had come to know her love, appreciate her warm hugs, enjoy her great sense of humor and laughter, and respect her spunkiness. As one of her children recently observed, "Augustine was like one of those Catholic saints she was in the habit of worshipping often. In fact, the Church ought to canonize her as another of their saints, because she had a specialness all to herself. None of us will ever forget her, because through all the generations of her extended family, she gave a great deal of love that will go on living forever in our hearts."

I became acquainted with this charming person through my Hispanic friend William Sandoval, who lives with his family on the same street, just down a few houses from where Augustine lived. She was his wife's relative, he told me, upon introducing us for the first time more than a year before Augustine's untimely demise. Although her eyesight was "a little worse for the wear" she still managed to get around quite well. In fact, I was surprised at just how nimble she appeared to be for someone her age.

There was *no evidence* whatsoever of any arthritis that I could discern from watching her movements. With someone interpreting for me, I asked this gallant lady why she didn't have any arthritis. Whereupon she managed a throaty laugh and replied in Spanish that it was because of *"dos remedios de hierbas medicinales,"* which had kept her totally free from painful swelling and tender joint inflammation all these many years.

To say that I was excited upon hearing it being attributed to "two remedies of medicinal herbs" is an understatement. I was ecstatic with joy and obviously quite eager to pump her for additional information, believing somewhere in the back of my mind that I might have actually stumbled onto a "secret cure" for the prevention, if not for the actual treatment, of arthritis itself!

Augustine hadn't managed to reach all these years without having acquired a fair amount of healing wisdom and some basic understanding of human nature as well. She was remarkably patient with this overanxious medical anthropologist, but teased my mind by *slowly* dribbling to me the information I wanted. I could tell there was no pressing or hurrying this old one, so I quietly resigned to taking down the data at her pace, which was somewhere between the speed of a slug and a snail. It took me *five hours,* several cups of tea, and a lot of in-between chit-chat on other subjects to obtain the data given here.

Augustine was born in the month of August (hence her name) in 1895 in Guadalupe, Colorado. Her mother Marcelina Valdez taught her much of what she knew about the use of herbs. Two plants, in particular, seemed to be her favorites. She made a tea from them that she had been faithfully drinking for nearly three quarters of a century. She also sometimes bathed in this same tea, soaking her body for 30 minutes or more in half a tub of hot water to which had been added *two quarts* of this hot tea.

By now my interest was at full peak and I was just getting ready to enjoy myself for the climax moment when she would reveal their identities to me. But, no, she suddenly, then and there, decided to show me pictures of *all* her grandchildren, great-grandchildren, and great-great grandchildren. Out came an entire photo gallery of nearly 100 kids. As she gave my interpreter and me the official "guided tour" through her family picture museum, she would pause and tell a little anecdote about this cute great-great grandson or that darling great-granddaughter.

If I ever needed my patience supplemented, it surely had to be on that occasion, for I had to call up a lot more of it from deep within my reservoirs of hidden virtues. And what astonished me even more was that I was able to manage some *genuine* smiles every now and then, while my brain sizzled and my stomach churned. But I got through the ordeal all right, however tortuous and arduous it may have appeared from my strangled perspective.

Augustine—bless her soul and may she rest in peace—*finally* got back to her discussion on herbs and picked up her former conversation on that subject remarkably well, without ever having missed a beat. The herbs that had kept her arthritis-free, she stated, were *epazote* and *escoba de la vibora*. After a puzzled look and a vocal expression of "Huh?" from me, she proceeded to pull out of her kitchen cupboard samples of both herbs to show me.

I recognized both of them right away. *Epazote* is another name for Mexican Tea *(Chenopodium ambrosioides)*. It is a rather scruffy-looking, nondescript *weed* that I've found growing in the sidewalk cracks of Hispanic barrios in Los Angeles, Barstow, Phoenix, and Albuquerque. In those places, though, it was usually a splayed-out, much trodden-on orphan, which indicated to me just how much low esteem it was held in by local residents.

The other plant is a small, many-stemmed, upright shrub with numerous narrow leaves and many little yellow flower clusters in bunches. The dried parts she showed me had an unmistakable resinous or waxy finish to them and when crushed gave off a slight piney odor. She spoke up, while handing me some of this *Escoba de la Vibora* (*Gutierrezia* or *Xanthocephalum* species): "This is an *insignificant* bush of *insignificant* height with *insignificant* leaves and flowers and about as uninteresting as a Mexican Chihuahua. To me it's only an *insignificant* tea that I drink *for the taste* and nothing more. I can't really understand why you should be showing it so much attention." At least, that's what my interpreter translated for me.

"Boy, is that ever the understatement of the century!" I thought to myself as I carefully surveyed samples of both herbs. Here I was, quite possibly looking at the "arthritis cure and preventive of the cen-

tury," and my informant had just dismissed one of the key ingredients rather casually by characterizing it as being "an *insignificant* little weed" of no real worth or value.

I recognized that both herbs were closely allied to other plants
with which I was also familiar. The epazote reminded me of lamb's
quarter *(Chenopodium album),* but lacking the other's lime-green, frost-
ed look. And escoba is equivalent to broomweed, growing on high and
dry slopes. mesas, bajadas, river bottoms, you name it, being the result
of overgrazing. *Both herbs are abundantly plentiful and very cheap to get.*

Augustine showed me how she made the tea, which she had been
drinking for most of her life. She filled an old tea kettle with what I
judged to have been a quart of water and set it on the stove to boil.
When it reached that stage, she added a small handful (probably about
two teaspoonsful) of *each* herb (or four teaspoonsful in all). This she let
simmer on low heat on a back stove burner for about 25 minutes before
removing it. When the tea had sufficiently cooled down to lukewarm,
she poured a cup out for each of us. I found to the tea to be just a tad
bitter, but a little addition of honey soon took care of that.

Augustine noted that she usually drank two cups of the stuff a
day, one in the morning while listening to an all-Spanish radio station and another cup in the evening while watching reruns of the old
"Lawrence Welk Show" on KBYU television. (Though she couldn't
understand the lyrics to the songs, she still loved to listen to the
music.) And about twice a week she would fill her tub half full of very
warm water and then add about two quarts of the hot tea and lie
down in it for a while to soak.

"I've never been in pain one day of my life since I've been doing
this," she said. From the looks of her physical activity, I had to con-
clude she was right. Ever since then, I've been recommending this, her
"secret remedy," to all those suffering from arthritis. Believe it or not, I
could almost do a separate book on that subject alone, having enough
testimonials from the hundreds who've tried it with great success.

Other Benefits: Good for Fungus, Ringworm, Intestinal Parasites, Sore Muscles, and Rheumatism

Augustine Gurule is with us no more, but her tea tonic is. And it has
a variety of other uses, being good for fungal infections, barber's itch,
athlete's foot, vaginitis, ringworm, tapeworm, roundworm, aching
muscles, tendonitis, and rheumatism. Use the tea internally and soak
the afflicted body part in some of the same liquid for up to 20 minutes at a time. You'll be surprised at just how effective it is for these
things.

ASTHMA/BRONCHITIS

Divinely Inspired Tea Remedy Saves Lives of Utah Herbalist and My Dad

The late German phytotherapist Rudolph Fritz Weiss, M.D., routinely recommended *warm* peppermint tea for some of his patients suffering from asthma or bronchitis. In the German edition of his best-selling book, *Lehrbuch der Phytotherapie* (Stuttgart: Hippokrates Verlag GmbH, 1985), he discussed what he thought were the some of the reasons for the herb's activity. He wrote that the volatile oil (0.7 percent), tannins (6 to 12 percent), and bitter principles interact with one another to strip unwanted mucus from the membrane linings of the lungs and expel them from the body. He noted that the volatile oil contained mostly menthol (between 50 and 60 percent), which he felt incorporated more oxygen into the respiratory system and helped unclog it.

Lobelia was the most controversial herb in American medicine during the early part of the 1800s. A man named Samuel Thomson, who claimed that God had inspired him with this remedy, put it at the center of an eclectic medical system bearing his name. Thomsonian medicine, as it later came to be called, relied heavily on lobelia. Doctors brave and open-minded enough to try lobelia on some of their patients discovered how wonderfully well it worked in the treatment of asthma, bronchitis, convulsions, diphtheria, laryngitis, and tonsillitis.

The muscle relaxant and antispasmodic activities were found mainly in the chief alkaloid lobeline, which exists primarily in the leaves and flowering tops of lobelia. In Thomson's time, American allopathic doctors undertook a vigorous campaign to destroy his system of natural medicine by labeling lobelia as a deadly poison. And in more recent times the Food and Drug Administration has declared lobelia, along with 26 other plants, as being "unsafe herbs." Most health food stores have removed the herb from their shelves, but it is still available from some herb companies by mail order. (You can get it from Great American Natural Products Inc., 4121 16th Street North, St. Petersburg, FL 33703; 800-323-4372.)

A Tea Remedy from Heaven

My father, Jacob Heinerman, was born January 5, 1914, in Salt Lake City, Utah. In 1996 he turned 82 years of age. He is able to breathe pretty well most of the time. But it wasn't always that way. For years, when my younger brother Joseph and I were growing up, our beloved dad suffered a lot from the symptoms of asthma.

Realizing the gravity of the situation at hand, he came to understand that unless he took some drastic action with this mounting health problem, his two young sons stood to become possible orphans. (Our mother had already died.)

Someone referred him to a practicing herbalist then working out of a tiny office between Second and Third West on First North in Provo, Utah. Because his own mother had used herbs a lot in the old country of Hungary, he felt comfortable going to see a man who used only natural remedies with which to heal.

The man's name was Dr. John Raymond Christopher, who later would become famous in his own right throughout much of North America as a premier herbalist. Ray, as he was called by those on intimate terms with him, was himself a walking "health miracle" of sorts. Years ago, while he was still actively lecturing for the National Health Federation at their many conventions, along with me and others, he took the time to tell me an extraordinary event from his own early childhood.

He said that while he was still very young he suddenly took sick with the croup one winter in Salt Lake City, where he then lived with his adoptive parents (his biological parents had abandoned him when he was born). Not knowing anything about the healing arts as such, his parents were panic stricken as to what to do for their son. Their anxieties were interrupted by a loud knock at the door.

One of them opened it to find an older man of medium build with an iron-gray beard standing in the cold without the benefit of a hat, coat, gloves, scarf, or boots to protect him from the intensely bitter weather. Yet, oddly enough, he wasn't shivering in the least bit. The stranger gave very explicit instructions on how to remove the congestion from the child's lungs and, thereby, stop his awful croup. The father listened attentively and then turned to ask his wife, who stood beside him, if she had heard everything, too. Then he turned back to the stranger to invite him inside, only to discover the man was gone. "There was *no* evidence of *any* footprints in that deep snow to ever indicate that someone had visited our home that night," I remember Ray telling me with deep soberness.

Ray's adoptive parents followed the instructions given them, and the boy was soon cured of his respiratory problem. Ray told me in that interview that he incorporated some of the elements of this divine cure in his own asthma remedy years later. And this is precisely what he prescribed to my father, when Jacob Heinerman visited him in his small office in Provo many years ago. He instructed my father to slowly *sip* a *warm* cup of peppermint tea into which had been put about 15 drops of tincture of lobelia. He promised his patient that this would help to expel most of the mucus clogging his bronchial tubes and allow him to breathe much more easily after that.

Ray also told my father to change his diet. He encouraged him to avoid all dairy products and sweets, for he believed that they contributed much to mucus-accumulating aspects of asthma. He also thought that the bleaching agents in white flour weren't good for the body either, and recommended that my dad switch to eating whole-grain breads and cereals. Dad followed this advice and noticed significant improvement after that.

AN INSPIRED REMEDY

$^2/_3$ cup fresh peppermint leaves, cut

OR

$^1/_2$ cup dried peppermint leaves

1 pint boiling water

Add the leaves, stir, cover with lid and set aside to steep for 20 minutes. Then add 15 drops lobelia tincture for every full cup of *warm* tea consumed. Take on an empty stomach preferably. If slight nausea sets in, eat a half slice of whole-wheat bread.

Here is how to make a lobelia tincture if you are unable to find one already made up. To make it, combine about one-half cup of powdered or cut lobelia leaves and flowers in one pint of good alcohol. Vodka, brandy, gin, or rum will all serve the same purpose. Shake every day, permitting the herb to extract for about 12 days. Let the botanical materials settle first before pouring off the tincture. Strain out the powder through a fine cloth, several layers of cheesecloth, or a clean paper coffee filter. Store the tincture in an amber bottle in a cool, dry place. Add *no more* than 15 drops per cup of *warm* peppermint tea. Sometimes, a *lesser* amount (10 drops) may be just as efficacious in the event that nausea sets in.

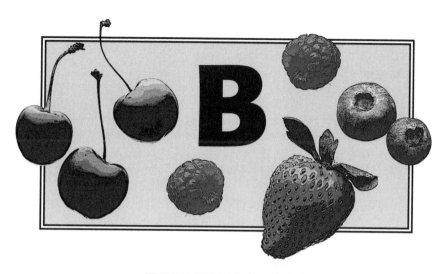

BACK STRAIN

Hot Tonic Packs and Refreshing Juices to Soothe Back Pain

THE PROBLEM

Back strain is a particular kind of terribly annoying pain caused by the overstretching or tearing of the back's supporting muscles. It seems to be most common in the thirty-something and over-forty crowd. At these ages back strength begins to diminish and people are more apt to abuse their backs.

Different things can produce back strain. The acute kind is often the result of improper movements or positioning for a common activity, such as sitting, bending, or lifting a heavy object. Speaking from my own experience, I know all too well how this can happen. I sit many hours of most days in my office at my old word processor, typing out a dozen or more pages of for my next health best-seller—as of the end of 1995 I was up to 43 titles and still counting! Unless I get up and walk around my research center and do some stretching exercises, I will usually develop an unpleasant crick in my neck or muscle spasm somewhere in my lower back. I suppose that's the price one pays for being well over six feet tall.

Back strain may, likewise, be induced by sudden trauma, such as an athletic injury. But more often than not, it usually occurs during routine activities.

Chronic back strain is most frequently precipitated by poor posture or poor conditioning and complicated by overuse, obesity, or pregnancy. Poor posture strains the lower back and makes it more vulnerable to injury. Weak and flabby abdominal muscles (for instance, "pot bellies" due to laziness, gluttony, and obesity) increase the risk of back strain. Aging also increases the risk of all types of back problems in general.

Back strain is one of the hardest things for doctors to correctly detect. Differential diagnosis of back pain can be unbelievably difficult, because it may also be caused by a wide variety of structural defects and systemic diseases. Unless the back pain clearly coincided with a wrenching movement or accident, diagnosis may involve a process of elimination more than anything else. Medical tests for observing such a thing could include X-rays and CT (computed tomography) and MRI (magnetic resonance imaging) scans.

The Solution

First, let's deal with some of the rather obvious things that can be done to treat a back strain. Resting whenever possible makes sense. Doing simple stretching exercises on the floor is another; Oriental and Indian exercises are good to do for this. They help to bring a measure of relief. Another thing is to lie down on a slant board for half an hour at a time.

Then there are the aquatic options: hot packs; soaking in a hot tub; taking a hot shower; or sitting in a Jacuzzi or whirlpool bath for a while. The first two are especially helpful in providing relief from back pain.

To make a nice herbal tonic for hot packs to be used on the back, boil a quart of *distilled* water. Set aside and add to it 7 drops each of oils of peppermint and eucalyptus. Stir with a wooden spoon, cover with a lid, and let sit for 10 minutes.

Lay a slant board on an angle; use a solid chair or some other piece of furniture for this. Do not angle it too high into the air—a two-foot elevation on one end is adequate for this. Or, it that isn't available, use an ironing board propped up the same way. If worse comes to worst, get a 3-foot-wide and 6-foot-long piece of ³/₄-inch interior plywood with a smooth side; lay the plywood down on the floor (at the angle described above) with the good side facing up.

Now uncover the pot of heated herbal liquid and with a pair of tongs insert a clean hand towel until it is thoroughly saturated. Using a wooden spoon, press the sides of the towel against the pot to remove excess liquid, so as not to make a mess on the floor. First, lay a large, *dry* bath towel over the slant board or plywood, then put this hot, wet hand towel in the center of the other towel. With the top part of your clothing removed, lie down so that your back is flat against this hot hand towel. It may be a good idea to throw a light blanket over your chest and hips to retain the heat as long as possible. It is critical when doing this to *move very quickly* to lie down, so that very little heat is lost in the process.

A much simpler way, though, if you have a friend or relative in your home with you is to have that person assist you. Remove your upper clothing and lie down flat on your stomach on the floor or a bed. Then have the other person dip the same hand towel into the pot and wring out any excess liquid as previously described. The wet towel is then placed over the bare back with a second, dry bath towel put on top to retain the heat. This process should be repeated every time the hand towel becomes cool to the skin. The treatment ought to last about half an hour. It is a great way to obtain immediate relief from back pain.

For soaking in a hot tub, fill it two thirds full of *pleasantly* hot (but not scalding) water. Then add about 20 drops of oils of peppermint or eucalyptus; mix well in the water by swishing back and forth with the hand. Gently ease yourself into the tub until your body is submerged almost up to your neck. Lie there for about 20 minutes enjoying the warm, relaxing feeling. You will be amazed at how quickly the pain of back strain can go away by doing this simple procedure.

Taking a hot shower can also help to some extent, but not quite the way a long soak in a hot tub of water can. For one thing, you don't have the benefit of the added herbal oils. For another, a shower wastes too much hot water for it to be of much good in the time that's needed.

Along with these aquatic procedures, there is another part of the program that I highly recommend, This should be done *just before* the hot pack or tub soak is started. It calls for drinking a very warm mug of special juice that will work from the inside to relieve muscle tension and nerve pain. You make the juice as follows:

BEEF AND BARLEY JUICE

1 medium carrot, cut in 1-inch pieces

1 celery rib, cut in 1-inch pieces

$1/_8$ cup barley, cooked

$1/_4$ cup onion

1 cup beef broth, boiling

pinch of cayenne pepper

pinch of granulated kelp

1 tsp. liquid Kyolic garlic

1. Place all ingredients in a Vita-Mix container (or equivalent food machine).
2. Secure the lid in place.
3. Move the black speed control lever to HIGH.
4. Lift the black lever to the ON position.
5. Run the machine for $3^1/_2$ minutes.
6. Makes two cups. Pour into a glass and drink.

Other Benefits: Helping Leg Cramp or "Charley Horse"

All of us at some time or another have gotten what is sometimes called a "Charley horse." This is nothing more than an old-fashioned leg cramp. The application of a hot pack in the form of a clean wash-cloth dipped into some of the hot herbal tonic previously mentioned, wrung out, and then put over the leg for a while will help to ease the pain considerably.

Get Rid of Chills and Shakes

During bouts of influenza, one of the most common symptoms is chills and shakes. Drinking one cup of the Beef and Barley Juice every few hours will help to allay this unpleasant sensation and make the body feel better.

BAD BREATH/BODY ODOR

What the Chinese Did for "Dragon Breath" and the Aztecs Did for "Goaty Armpits"

THE PROBLEM

What we're dealing with here is a *single* problem, but emitted from two different parts of the body. The matter at hand is a bad smell coming from the mouth and from beneath the arms.

A lot of people are bothered with halitosis. A variety of factors can be at work here to produce "dragon breath." It may be due to poor dental hygiene; insufficient brushing and flossing of the teeth and regular rinsing of the mouth will leave food particles trapped inside, which soon decay and cause a smell. Also, gum disease, tooth decay, nasal infection, or a sore throat will usually produce a rank aroma.

Diet certainly has a lot to do with halitosis. The wrong combination of foods, consumed at any given time, is bound to be a factor in all this. A green chili enchilada and a medium-sized Coke or a large pepperoni pizza will do the trick here. So will chewing a clove of raw garlic or eating a meal laced with lots of onions; but, at the very least, these spices are good for you, even if their odors aren't.

The smoking of a cigar, cigarette, or pipe will make the mouth smell something like the chimney of a mountain cabin in which has been recently burned some type of hard-wood logs. Or, perhaps, such smokers' mouths may remind others of car exhaust fumes. Either way, the breath is quite disgusting.

The inadequate chewing of food may also contribute to bad breath. Meals that are hurriedly gulped down tend to get only half digested as a rule. The unfortunate results are the commencement of an internal fermentation with some of the nasty odors spewing up the gullet and out of the mouth. Not to mention the constipation such careless eating habits produce; as food wastes accumulate in the bowels, gases tend to travel *upward,* besides outward, producing stink at *both* ends.

Body odor may sometimes be linked with poor digestion, liver malfunction, bowel irregularity, and excessive meat consumption. The toxic wastes generated from consumed animal flesh find their way out of the body through the pores of the skin. When I was in the funeral business many years ago, working for a period of time at Berg Mortuary in Provo, Utah, I learned early on in the business which corpses had been meat eaters and the very few who had been vegetarian for most of their lives. Whenever we went to pick up the remains of a deceased person that had been lying around for several hours the unmistakable presence of methane gas was easily detected by our olfactory senses—except in a few cases, where the corpses hardly smelled at all, even after being lifeless for some hours before they were discovered. Wondering as to why this was so, we inquired of friends or relatives who were there when we arrived for our pick-ups, and invariably found the dead people to have practiced a vegetarian lifestyle for a number of years.

A second primary source for body odor is ofttimes poor hygiene. What a difference a little soap and water and some light scrubbing of the body can do for changing the smell of the body. Bacteria tend to breed on the surface of the skin all the time and need to be washed away quite often; when this doesn't happen, their numbers rapidly accumulate. We may not be able to see them because they are so tiny and invisible to the naked eye; but, boy, can we ever smell their presence on someone else from just a few feet away!

Another consideration for body odor, which can't be helped with any of the juices, teas, or tonics mentioned in this book is the possession of a mortal tabernacle by one or more evil spirits. I'll admit that it sounds a bit hokey, but upon more careful reflection makes sense: When I was a young boy growing up in Provo, my father owned and operated The Cottage Book Shop, located at 177 North 100 East. We lived in a large Victorian-style house with huge rooms and high ceilings. The parlor, drawing room, dining room, and living room contained the book shop, while our small family of three resided in the back kitchen, pantry, bathrooms, and assorted bedrooms.

Just down the street south of us by one block was Speckert's Market. "Old man Speckert," as the kids in the neighborhood not so fondly called him, was a crotchety, frowning, middle-aged man with the most cantankerous disposition of anyone I'd ever encountered in my youth. I had to make frequent trips there for groceries and, to this day, can still vividly remember the *peculiar odor* this man carried with him always. I wasn't due to poor hygiene by any means, for he kept himself immaculately clean, well groomed, and nicely attired at all times. Once, I asked my wise father why "old man Speckert" smelled so bad. My father, first of all, corrected me by saying that it wasn't nice to call him an "old man," but to refer to him as "Mr. Speckert." Then he gave as his opinion the possibility that this man, for some unknown reasons, was possessed with evil spirits, which my dad sincerely believes to this day, and that this was the cause of the grocery man's weird smell!

I know that this train of logic seems rather subjective and even judgmental to some. But when I became an adult and began surveying the world around me and the wonderful variety of people in it, I was more inclined to think my father's assessment correct than to dispute it.

The Solution

The ancient Chinese and Aztecs had some simple solutions for the problems they characterized as "dragon breath" and "goaty armpits." The Orientals have always *nibbled* on some aniseed or small pieces of *raw* ginseng or licorice root to get rid of bad breath. They also thought that the liver needed resuscitating or the bowels moved often to rectify the situation. Dandelion root tea was routinely prescribed for the former and the consumption of certain *fresh* fruits (or their juices) for the latter.

The tea was made by cooking one-half handful of cleaned dandelion root in one pint of water, covered, for 15 minutes. Then the tea was cooled, strained, and a cup or more consumed. To evoke a nice bowel movement, a handful of any *fresh* berries, one-half or a whole melon, a small cucumber, or 10 lychee nuts would be eaten slowly.

The Aztecs, on the other hand, took a more practical approach to the problem of "goaty armpits." Rather than thinking it might have been something of an *internal* nature causing the smell, they employed simple remedies for external use only. I use as my source for this the scholarly work entitled the *Florentine Codex: General History of the Things of New Spain* by Fray Bernardino de Sahagún and translated from the Ancient Aztec into English, with appropriate footnotes by Charles E. Dibble and Arthur J.O. Anderson (Santa Fe: The School of American Research and The University of Utah, 1963; Number 14, Part XII, Book 11, pertaining to "Earthly Things").

Consider this one solution for "goaty armpits":

[Original Aztec]

Vei Vauhqujlitl, Anoço Teuvauhqujlitl, chichic: vauhtli piltontli, tepiton: in ie vei vel chichic, paoaxonj.

[Modern English]

Uei Uauhquilitl or Teouauhquilitl
It is bitter. It is young, small amaranth. When mature, it is very bitter. Crush on rock and rub juice beneath arms.

For those who may need to know something about it, amaranth is an erect annual, some 1 to 6 feet high, and branched above. Another name by which it is commonly known is pigweed. The stemmed leaves, about 3 to 6 inches long, are a rather dull green, rough, hairy, ovate, or rhombic, with wavy rims. The small flower clusters end in pyramidal, loosely branched, reddish or greenish inflorescences. The fleshy taproots, lengthy and pinkish to red in color, also have medicinal properties to them. From a nutritional standpoint, it is equal to parsley in iron, chlorophyll, and water contents. In fact, parsley is sometimes listed as a major ingredient in natural chlorophyll-based body deodorants found in many health food stores.

Since pigweed grows just about anywhere, it can be used for removing body odor. The best time to pick it is in the spring and early summer when much of its moisture content still remains; as the summer and fall progress, the plant tends to dry out more, thus making it unfit to use for this purpose. Cut up enough pigweed into small pieces to equal one-half cup. Put this into a food blender or Vita-Mix unit, barely add just enough water (maybe $1/4$ cup), and turn on for $1^1/_2$ minutes. The resulting liquid should be somewhat thick, but not mushy. If too thick, add a little more water and blend again to dilute it. Pour into a small dish. Use several cotton balls held together and dip into some of the pigweed juice and apply thoroughly beneath each armpit. Use a hair dryer to dry more quickly, if necessary. And don't worry about turning the skin or armpit hairs green; the stain isn't permanent and will easily wash off with soap and water when showering later on.

For those readers who may by a little reluctant or timid to try something green under their armpits, how about another ancient Aztec remedy, which I *know* for a fact *works great,* but won't turn your skin the color of the Jolly Green Giant's? The ancient Mexicans called it tlilxochitl. They took the cured pods and liquefied them by hand, then rubbed some of this tlilxochitl beneath their arms to get rid of this "goaty" smell. I decided to try this once for myself. I poured a little bit ($1/_2$ teaspoon) of commercially available tlilxochitl into a cup, dipped several cotton balls into it, and rubbed the scented solution under each armpit. The pleasant aroma lasted for hours and didn't even give me a rash as regular colognes have done.

I bet by now you're anxiously awaiting the English translation of tlilxochitl—would you believe, if I told you, that it was ordinary pure *vanilla* extract? That's right, "a spice that's nice, for underarm smell the goats can tell."

Other Benefits: Treatment for Bleeding, Anemia, Inflammation, Sores, and Wounds

Fresh amaranth juice is wonderful for treating a variety of other health problems. In a food blender or Vita-Mix unit, combine 1 cup of fresh amaranth (which has been cut into small pieces) with 3 ice cubes and 1 cup *warm* water. This should produce a nice green liquid that is of mild temperature. Drink it straight or mix in some tomato or carrot juice. It has enough iron to reverse anemia (if taken regularly for several months), can stop internal hemorrhaging, and reduce swelling and inflammation.

Soak some cotton balls in a little bit of this amaranth juice and bathe sores or wounds. Do this several times each day and watch just how quickly the skin begins to heal itself.

A Natural Tranquilizer

For those suffering from nervousness, stress, hypertension, or hyperactivity, there is something else to consider besides the standard herbal remedies like chamomile, skullcap, and valerian. A warm cup of *distilled* water to which have been added 8 drops of pure vanilla extract and slowly sipped as well as *savored* by the nostrils will have such a calming effect upon the system that it will surprise you.

BALDNESS

What a Japanese Sumo Wrestler Does for His Male-Pattern Baldness

DESCRIPTION

Tea drinking originated in China several thousand years ago. The Chinese name for it is *ch'a,* but it is the South China dialect version of *t'e* that undoubtedly gave birth to our modern equivalent of *tea*—originally pronounced "tay" in seventeenth-century England.

A knowledge of tea entered Japan around the eighth century, long before it was exported from China to Europe. The Japanese adopted the standard Chinese name but customarily place their *cha* with an honorific *o.* This conveniently distinguishes their "green" tea from *kōcha,* the name given to the "black" tea drunk almost everywhere else in the world, as well as in Japan itself. It is an added irony that in two island nations, England and Japan—located half a world apart from each other—that this Chinese beverage should have taken its strongest hold.

In England the tea ritual is a deep-seated part of the daily cultural routine, bordering nearly on religious status. The old adage, "To separate an Englishman from his 'spot of tea,' is to invoke the wrath of the Queen," perhaps holds more truth than meets the eye. On the other hand, in Japan, tea *is* a religion, in fact the very vehicle of the spiritual discipline of Zen Buddhism's *chadō,* the Way of Tea, not to mention being an indispensable part of everyday life there.

What Makes Tea Either "Green" or "Black"?

Japanese tea is 'green," whereas the teas of China and India and the type that is usually drunk in the West are "black." With very few variations in agricultural techniques, the tea bushes in Japan are identical to those found growing in the shadow of the mighty Himalayas. What makes Japanese tea green and the other Asian teas black is how each one is processed.

In Japan, once tea leaves are picked, they are immediately steamed. If tea is not given this treatment, an enzyme in the leaf ferments and the leaves turn black. The steaming process is one the Indians and Sri Lankans don't adhere to. But if the enzyme is destroyed through steaming, the leaves stay green; this, in turn, make green tea.

Male-Pattern Baldness Glorified

Medical statistics show that 50 percent of Caucasian males have experienced some noticeable male-pattern baldness by the time they reach age 50. Only 37 percent of postmenopausal women, however, show some evidence of hair loss. Alopecia is believed to be mostly hereditary.

But some men have been able to capitalize on their hair loss and have even made it part of their appearance trademarks. No two better examples of alopecia come to mind than Yul Brynner and Telly Savalas, both of whom are now deceased. The former won an Academy Award some years ago for his outstanding portrayal of the defiant and arrogant young ruler in the film classic *The King and I*. Savalas, who suffered from a medical hair-loss condition clinically known as cicatricial alopecia, became instantly recognizable to millions of television viewers as the bald New York City police detective who loved to suck on lollipops in the hit series *Kojak*.

Both men helped to deemphasize the presumed shame and embarrassment that usually accompanies many cases of early male-pattern baldness. They turned an obvious problem into great success for themselves and certainly conveyed a more positive image to American males about baldness in general. In fact, I remember some years ago watching Savalas on a late-night talk show and hearing him remark to the program host and audience: "Hey, baby! Bald is beautiful and don't you forget it!" At the same time he gave the top of his head an affectionate rub with his hand.

Hair Restoration Secrets of a Japanese Sumo Wrestler

A few years ago I had occasion to travel to the "Land of the Rising Sun" in company with some other folks from different countries, such as Denmark, England, Germany, America, New Zealand, and Australia. We were the specially invited guests of Wakunaga Pharmaceutical Company, makers of the world's premier selling, best-researched, and most effective garlic product, sold under the trade name of Kyolic.

We went to many cities and met lots of interesting people. Among those I was fortunate to meet was a well-known Japanese sumo wrestler whose name has since escaped my memory. I was introduced to him through one of our capable interpreters. This man was awesome in size and proportion, weighing in at a whopping 303 pounds. And yet, I was reliably informed by our interpreter that he was considered one of the *"skinny"* kids on the block, with other wrestlers outweighing him by as much as 100 or 200 pounds *more!*

I asked this near-naked potential candidate for a Jenny Craig or Nutri/System weight-loss program how he was able to put on so much weight. His reply was one word, *"Chankonabe!"* This is the traditional stew of fish and vegetables that all sumo wrestlers consume in hefty portions. My interpreter and I accompanied our huge host to one of several *chanko* shops in the Ryogoku district in the middle of Tokyo's older working-class section. Here we chowed down with our friend a typical *chanko* meal. The one we had that day consisted of crab, clam, salmon, sardines, scallops, beef, chicken, and vegetables, all cooked in a pot over a gas grill in the middle of our table. He ate ten times as much as we did!

I noticed that this former *yokozuna* or grand champion and previous winner of the huge silver Emperor's Cup had a nice, thick head of long, black hair done up into a bun near the back on top of his head. Some of the other wrestlers we had met before were showing signs of encroaching hair loss near the tops of their foreheads. But this clearly wasn't the case with our friend. So I asked him in between mouthfuls what he did to prevent *early* male-pattern baldness.

His answer astonished me. He said that every morning upon arising (usually at about 5:30 A.M.), he made for himself a small pot of green tea. After letting it cool a bit, he would then sponge some of it onto his head while sitting on a wooden bench with his body slightly bent over a large pan on the floor. He would then commence massaging his entire scalp very vigorously with all his fingers.

The usual method would be for him to begin above his forehead and push all the way back toward the neck. Then, with his fingers still spread apart, he would pull them back over the scalp again to where he started. He went back and forth in this direction about seven times, always sponging some more *warm* green tea into his hair before doing so. After this he changed the position of his hands, this time placing them over the ears with the fingers still spread apart. He would then push upward toward the center of the crown until his fingertips met and would then pull them back down again toward the ears. He did this for about the same number of times.

There would be about $2^1/_2$ cups of green tea remaining, which he would then drink before commencing his morning workout in the ring knocking heads with other sumos. He said that this thing had been in his father's family for several generations and that everyone who used it *never* became bald. He also let it be known through our interpreter that it would *not* work where baldness had already been established for some time.

Perfect Digestive Aid

Our big friend with the flaps of rolling flesh had an aura of dignity about him, in spite of being a fierce and tough warrior inside the *dohyo* or hard-clay ring. This nobility of spirit is known in Japanese as *hinkaku* and embraces everything that is worthy and of good report.

This fellow wrestled with some 31 others in the top *makunouchi* division. During several of his workout sessions with other behemoths, it dawned on me what sumo really is all about. It's a power thing, pure and simple. I mean, here you have two human elephants pushing, shoving, flailing, and grunting at each other inside a small ring that I'd estimate to be no more than about 15 feet in diameter.

After giving one opponent a hard shove, which knocked him on his backside, our friend stepped outside the *dohyo* and wiped the sweat off his face with a wet towel. We joined him again for another enormous meal. I wanted to know if this guy ever got indigestion from eating so much. Our interpreter posed the question, and my sumo friend laughed heartily. He shook his head and replied that he *never* suffered from indigestion of any kind so long as he drank plenty of green tea with his meals. He claimed it was the best digestive aid for heavy eating.

BREWING GREEN TEA, SUMO STYLE

There are a number of ways to brew green or black tea. But here is the one preferred by many of Japan's great sumo wrestlers.

1. Select a teapot made of china, earthenware, glass, silver, or stainless steel.

2. Rinse the teapot out with boiling water (to heat it) and dry it thoroughly.

3. Place 6 teabags of green tea inside the pot.

4. Then pour 6 cups of boiling water over them. *Never* heat a teapot directly on the stove, as it will completely ruin the flavor and effectiveness of the tea you're making.

5. Cover the teapot and let its contents steep between 8 and 12 minutes. My sumo friend stated with some obvious pride that he like to brew his tea for 15 minutes, which gave it a stronger flavor.

6. Strain the tea and let it cool down a little before drinking lukewarm.

BENIGN PROSTATIC HYPERTROPHY (BPH)

(see under Prostate Problems)

BLADDER INFECTION

Tonic Juices and Herbal Therapy for Infected Men and Women

DESCRIPTION

In one of my other national best-sellers in this health book series, *Heinerman's Encyclopedia of Nuts, Berries, and Seeds* (Englewood Cliffs NJ: Prentice Hall, 1995), I point out that "all berries . . . are rich in many different trace elements." It is these micronutrients that enable the immune system to actively combat whatever bacterial infection may be lurking in the bladder. Berries also contain ellagic acid, which assists the body in fighting infection, especially when it comes to cancer of the bladder.

Certain water-holding fruits and vegetables such as melons, cucumbers, and tomatoes should always be consumed in great abundance when bladder infection is suspected. Because of their high moisture content, they are able to actually flush out infectious bacteria that may be adhering to any parts of the bladder.

Carrot, garlic, and onion contain important nutrients that have antibiotic properties. The beta-carotene in carrots and the sulfur amino acids in both allium species are clearly antibacterial and antiviral in how they work against infections of all kinds.

The acidic quality of the vinegar makes it more difficult for harmful bacteria to remain in the system for very long. And the medical evidence in support of vitamin C has shown how well it works against infection.

A number of medicinal herbs have certain constituents in them that help the body to resist invasion by unfriendly bacteria or harmful viruses. Goldenseal, for instance, contains the important alkaloids hydrastine, hydrastinine, and berberine, which have proven to be very effective against the bacteria E. coli and Staphylococcus aureus. Juniper berry extract has been tested in various cell cultures and found to be very useful against cancer, influenza virus A2, and herpes simplex virus I and II. Peppermint contains a volatile oil composed mainly of menthol, menthone, and menthyl acetate. This trio of compounds is responsible for the herb's antiviral activities against Newcastle disease, herpes simplex, vaccinia, Semliki Forest, and West Nile viruses in egg and cell-culture systems.

Finally, international research has demonstrated that honey is an effective weapon against infection, too. An Israeli research team headed by Dr. Arieh Bergman published its findings to this effect in a report entitled, "Acceleration of Wound Healing by Topical Application of Honey," which appeared in the *American Journal of Surgery* (Vol. 145, March 1983.) It noted that "honey is hypertonic and has been shown to be sterile and highly bactericidal." Infectious wounds treated with honey were smaller and the "depth of tissue repair was greater." A French scientist, Yves Donadieu, read a paper entitled "The Use of Honey in Natural Therapeutics" before the Apitherapy Second Symposium held in Romania in the mid-1970s. He found that "honey increases resistance [to disease] and helps strengthen the [immune system]."

Multiple Therapies for Infected Bladders

Two of the simplest and most immediate measures which can be taken to help treat bladder infection are:

1. The *increased* consumption of water. Doctors believe that such hydration is good for helping to flush out some of this gram negative bacteria from the urinary tract.

2. The discontinuance of sexual activity until the problem is cured. Most urologists are convinced that routine acts of sex tend only to prolong bladder infection.

After these things come other alternatives. A change in what a person eats and drinks is essential to keeping a proper acid-base balance in the body. Moreover, alternative-minded physicians seem to think that by *increasing* the acid content of the urine, it can help to retard bacterial growth. To achieve this, an individual must cut back on his or her intake of whole grain products, cereals, milk, cheese, and butter for up to three weeks. And during this same period a *minimum* of most fruits and vegetables should also be consumed until improvement is noticed.

But what can be taken in generous amounts are most berries and berry juices. Whole strawberries and raspberries, when in season and available, should be consumed with gusto. Ditto, likewise, for blackberry and cranberry juice; as much as 2–3 glasses a day of either can be beneficial for the body. In fact, a number of studies involving cranberry juice have appeared in the medical literature over the last two and a half decades showing how valuable cranberry juice is for clearing up bladder infection.

Different kinds of melons (crenshaw, honeydew, and cantaloupe), including watermelon, are very good additions to a limited recovery diet and should be eaten with enthusiasm. Fresh cucumbers are an added bonus, too.

A combination of $1/3$ beet and $2/3$ carrot or tomato juice are worthy vegetable tonics to be drinking. However, their *acidity* needs to be *increased* before drinking them. Adding one tablespoon of liquid Kyolic garlic or a teaspoon of yellow onion juice to an 8-fluid-ounce glass of either juice combination will accomplish this purpose. Or one can simply add 2 teaspoons of apple cider vinegar to the same concoctions to boost their acidity more. When more acidic liquid passes through the bladder, the infectious bacterial count substantially decreases, whereas with high alkalinity in the blood the bacteria thrive and multiply like crazy.

Megadoses of vitamin C are always good to take for such problems. I would suggest somewhere between 6,000 and 12,000 milligrams in acute cases. These amounts can be cut in half when improvement becomes evident. Vitamin A intake should be as much as 50,000 units a day in the beginning, but tapering off to about 20,000 IU as a maintenance dose. I would urge, however, that *fish oil* capsules of A be used instead of vegetable-derived beta-carotene (another form of A).

Herbs to be taken with any of the foregoing juices mentioned should include goldenseal root in capsule form (two a day), unless you happen to be hypoglycemic. If that is the case, then switch to juniper or cedar berries (three capsules daily). Use these herbs for *no more* than three weeks at a time with a two-week interval of discontinuance.

Warm peppermint tea is very good for bladder infection, especially when some honey is added (1 tablespoon per cup of tea) to increase the acidity. Boil a pint of water and add $1/2$ cup dried peppermint leaves. Cover with lid and set aside to steep for 20 minutes. Strain, reheat if necessary, add the honey, and drink.

Rinses out Blood Impurities

One of the definite advantages of eating fresh berries in season or drinking various berry juices is that they help to flush out accumulated toxins from the system. Think of berries in terms of a rinsing action, because that pretty much is how they work chemically to purify the blood.

Constipation Cleared up

An old traditional remedy from the Ozark Mountains has been the use of fresh blackberries or their juice for promoting a healthy bowel movement in case the colon is plugged up. I've had a number of mountain folk informants tell me so in past years. And I've tried it on occasion for myself to discover just how quickly a laxative effect can be evoked with blackberries.

On the other hand, a tea made from blackberry leaves and roots is a long-standing solution for diarrhea. Cook 1 teaspoon each of leaves and root in 1 pint of water on low heat, covered, for 12 minutes. Take $1/_2$ cup *cool* tea every $1^1/_2$ hours or as needed.

Methods of Application

Water. Tap water high in chlorine content, while not good for our overall health, is, nevertheless, quite useful for eradicating bladder infections. So, too, is spring or mineral water. The chlorine and other elements in them help to destroy the bacteria causing the problem.

Juices. Here are some inventive but practical juice recipes for strengthening the function of the bladder. They work more quickly and effectively because they're consumed in liquid form and don't have to be subjected to the usual ways things are routinely eaten and digested.

BERRY POWDER DRINK

$1/_2$ cup cold cranberry juice

$1/_2$ cup cold blackberry juice

$1/_4$ cup whole cranberry sauce

$1/_3$ cup frozen strawberries

$1/_3$ cup frozen raspberries

2 tsp. honey

$2/_3$ cup ice cubes

Place all ingredients in a Vita-Mix Total Nutrition Center container or equivalent food machine in the order given. Secure the complete 2-part lid by locking under the tabs. Move the black speed control level to HIGH. Then lift the black lever to the ON position and allow the unit to run for $1^1/_2$ minutes, until everything is smooth. Makes about $1^3/_4$ cups.

Vegetable Surprise

Here is a nifty vegetable tonic that will boost the powers of your immune system to an astonishing degree. Not only is it good for bladder infection, but it is of equal value in treating just about any other problem in the body that is caused by unfriendly bacteria or harmful viruses. But it works more efficiently when taken *hot!*

> $1^1/_2$ *cups water, boiling*
>
> $^1/_2$ *cucumber, unpeeled*
>
> $^1/_2$ *cup tomatoes, fresh or canned*
>
> $^1/_8$ *cup sauerkraut, canned or homemade*
>
> $^1/_4$ *cup carrots*
>
>   *2 tbsp. liquid Kyolic garlic (see Product Appendix)*
>
>   *1 tbsp. fresh onion*
>
>   *juice from half of a cut lemon, manually squeezed into the container*
>
> $^1/_4$ *tsp. Mrs. Dash*
>
> $^1/_2$ *tsp. Worcestershire sauce*
>
>   *1 tsp. apple cider vinegar*

Place all the above ingredients in the Vita-Mix container or equivalent food machine in the order listed. Follow the rest of the instructions given in the previous recipe. Run the machine for $2^1/_2$ minutes until contents are smooth. Makes almost 2 cups. Drink while still very warm.

BLOOD CLOTS

How a Former American Vice-President Might Have Been Saved from a Life-Threatening Medical Situation with Herbal Tonics

DESCRIPTION

Cayenne pepper contains a volatile compound called capsaicin. Ginger root contains an oily resin called gingerol. Garlic contains a wide assortment of sulfur compounds. And cold-water fish such as salmon, mackerel, menhaden, herring, and sardines have a high fat content in their oils and provide more omega-3 fatty factors than other fishes.

All these items do one thing in the body—they prevent blood clots from occurring. Clots are formed when blood cells become exceedingly sticky and commence bunching together. But the afore-mentioned compounds do away with this stickiness, which stops the "grape-clustering effect" so that blood cells can continue sliding over one another more easily.

How Herbs Could Have Solved Dan Quayle's Health Problems

During 1994 former U.S. Vice-President Dan Quayle of Indiana was giving serious consideration to throwing his hat into the 1995 polit-ical arena and making a run for the office of U.S. president. His advis-ers said he had a very good chance of winning the Republican nom-ination because of his youthful appeal, tremendous charisma, and seemingly boundless energy.

But what he hadn't counted on derailing these plans was the proverbial "monkey wrench," which came in the form of an itty bitty little substance known medically as an embolism. A blood clot formed in one of the large veins of the former vice-president's legs. Soon a piece of that blood clot broke off, roaming through his system back toward the heart. From there it traveled into the pulmonary arteries, the blood vessels going directly to his lungs.

Had he not received the prompt emergency medical attention that he did, chances are he might have died. But when medics rolled him into an Indianapolis hospital on the night of November 28, 1994, he was promptly given an intravenous injection of heparin. This well-known drug quickly starts to "thin" the blood to prevent further blood clots from forming.

However, three common kitchen spices could have worked just as well had the former vice-president taken them well in advance. They are cayenne pepper, ginger root, and garlic. Although he undoubtedly knew of their association with food preparation, he was woefully ignorant of their marvelous medicinal virtues. And this because, like so many millions of other Americans, he had been raised in the traditions of his parents to rely solely on medical doctors, drugs, and surgery, if necessary, for help with health problems.

But I know of an individual who is the same age as Mr. Quayle, not to mention being very close to him in height, weight, and physical build. However, he has grown up in an environment completely different from that which Dan Quayle did. This man was raised in a tradition of home remedies, where herbs were just as natural to take as aspirin might be for someone else.

This individual put himself on a simple supplemental program using herbal tonics in 1989. But like Mr. Quayle, my friend didn't exercise very much and was under a lot of stress, though his job wasn't at all connected to politics. My friend spared himself an embolism like the one that nearly killed Indiana's favorite son.

Blood Clot-Busting Tonic

Here is the tonic my friend took on a regular basis to keep from getting a blood clot. He claims that "a little bit goes a long way" toward warding off potential, life-threatening embolisms. He says drinking the stuff straight is only for "real he-men or female Amazons" who don't mind some "fire and action" in the taste of whatever they're drinking at the time. All others, he insists, should use tomato or V-8 juice as "chasers" for this lively little number, because of its overpowering effects on the senses.

> $1/_2$ **cup canned salmon, mackerel, or sardines**
>
> $1/_2$ **cup canned tomatoes or tomato juice or V-8 juice**
>
> **2 tbsp. fresh, grated ginger root**
>
> **1 clove garlic, peeled**
>
> $1/_4$ **tsp. powdered cayenne pepper**

Place all these ingredients in a Vita-Mix Total Nutrition Center container or equivalent food blender in the order given. Secure the lid and turn speed control knob to HIGH. Then flip the lever to the ON position and run the unit for $1^1/_2$ minutes, until everything comes out smooth. Makes a little over one cup.

NOTE: Sometimes my friend likes to add 2–3 tablespoons of Teriyaki sauce, two raw oysters, and $1/_2$ cup ice cubes for what he describes as "an interesting variation to an already unusual drink."

BREAST CANCER

Juice Tonics for Women to Take to Avoid Getting Breast Cancer

DESCRIPTION

In spite of all the marvelous technological advances made in modern medicine within recent years, doctors are still very much in the dark as to exactly what causes breast cancer. Two popular and recent medical references consulted by large numbers of doctors offer no explanation as to its origins. *The 5-Minute Clinical Consult* by Drs. H. Winter Griffith and Mark R. Dambro (Philadelphia; Lea & Febiger, 1994; p. 16) lists "Unknown" beside the category marked CAUSES in heavy, bold type under the entry of Breast Cancer. And the *Johns Hopkins Symptoms and Remedies* (New York: Rebus, 1995; p. 358), put out by America's best overall hospital of the same name, made this terse comment under its DISORDERS section for Breast Cancer: "The precise cause is unknown . . . ."

So it appears, even from the most reliable medical literature currently available, that doctors still don't have a single clue as to what might possibly cause the most common cancer among women today. But if you're a woman reading these words, I'd like to offer a point of view that contradicts this other "we-don't-know" position. The concept is radical and the ideas behind it totally revolutionary, but by any means the theories about to be advanced are grounded firmly in *solid science* and not just mere speculation.

Yes, Virginia, there *is,* indeed, an explanation for the causes of breast cancer. To look for it, however, one must go into something called Darwinian medicine. It began back sometime in 1980 when the world's leading expert on how infectious diseases originate, Dr. Paul Ewald of Amherst College in Massachusetts, proposed using Charles Darwin's controversial theory of evolution to illuminate the beginnings of certain symptoms of infectious diseases. Now, well into the close of this century, he's become a major force behind what some are touting as the next great medical upheaval: the application of Darwin's ideas pertaining to natural selection in attempting to understand how human diseases came into being.

First of all, you need to believe in evolution to some extent. I don't mean the radical kind that says we all came from monkeys, but the more-common sense approach that suggests that everything evolves from something simple into something more complex.

Next, you need to realize that even though you might be a nineties type of woman—independent, free-thinking, self-willed, and career-motivated—you're still chained to a body designed for the Stone Age. Think of it another way. Your ancestral body belonged to the Pliocene times, where many thousands of years ago you prepared and cooked the saber-toothed tigers that your hairy cave husband brought home after each hunting trip. You got lots of exercise, lived outdoors a great deal, and all that sort of stuff. But now your present body probably sits in front of a computer screen in a corporate office in a midtown high-rise somewhere. And for much of the day the only exercise you get is playing with a mouse. Over long eons of time your body biochemistry has changed in all sorts of unknown ways.

Evolutionary biologists like Ewald and medical anthropologists like myself are now proposing that some of these biochemical changes are behind today's breast cancer epidemic. While it's obviously quite impossible to study a prehistoric woman's biochemistry, there are still groups of hunter-gatherers around—like the San of Africa—who make admirable stand-ins for the real thing.

Scientists such as ourselves have made professional careers out of studying these types of modern Stone Age societies. As a result we've learned many astonishing things that are slowly turning the medical world upside down in terms of how some doctors are beginning to view the disease process. It has been my own experience among such prehistoric cultures to find the biochemistries of these women at great variances with their counterparts in urban life.

A foraging lifestyle is a lifestyle in which the average menstruation begins *later*. Among such women the first child is usually born *earlier* and there are invariably *more* children overall per female. And breast feeding is marked more in *years* than in months (as is commonly the case now). I've also noticed that menopause often comes somewhat *earlier* in life.

By comparing all these natural observations with today's liberated American women, it isn't difficult at all to see how breast cancer came about. Women in the United States at present probably experience 3.5 times *more* menstrual cycles than their ancestors did 15,000 years ago. During each cycle a woman's body is flooded with the hormone estrogen. And breast cancer, as clinical research has found, is very much estrogen related. The more frequently the breasts are exposed to the hormone, the greater the chance that a tumor will take hold. In fact, women today are somewhere between 10 and 100 times more apt to be stricken with breast cancer than their Stone Age relatives were, depending, of course, on whose data you're following.

Returning Your Body's Biochemistry to Stone Age Standards

Now that you understand how breast cancer (along with a multitude of other diseases) most likely came about, you need some valuable information on how to *reverse* those biochemical changes that evolved into our bodies over a lengthy time. Bear in mind that the suggestions given here won't keep you completely free of breast cancer; but, at least, they will substantially *lower* your risk of ever contracting it in your lifetime.

My first suggestion is that you start *walking* more often. Women in prehistoric times did a lot of it, and so should you. Walking is the finest way I know of to balance the circulation. When a woman sits too much, she soon accumulates toxins in her body-tissue fat. But with every step taken, her lymphatic system is gently massaged. This movement helps return the two quarts of fluid that are stashed away in places like the breasts to the central circulation where they can be processed, purified, and returned full of vigor and vitality.

Walking is *the* preferred form of exercise among the hunting-gathering societies with whom I've spent some time in the past. It is not running or pumping iron, but simple strolling. Modern-day women who enjoy doing heavy workouts in the gym or classroom may, in fact, be exposing themselves to a *greater* risk of breast cancer than if they didn't exercise at all. As fantastic as this statement seems, it has some pretty sound clinical research to back it up. Kenneth Cooper, M.D., the "father of aerobics," who once encouraged unlimited exercise, now has revised his thinking on the matter. In a controversial book he recently wrote, *Dr. Kenneth H. Cooper's Antioxidant Revolution* (Nashville: Thomas Nelson Publishers, 1994) he sensibly argues *too much* vigorous exercise could lead to the development of cancer in men and women. Exercise, as he correctly points out, unleashes small armies of marauding free radicals which are linked to cancer throughout the body. Walking, though, is the *only* low-intensity, stress-free exercise that puts *minimal* amounts of these aberrant molecules into the system.

The next thing that needs to be done to return your body's biochemistry to Stone Age standards is to learn *correct* breathing. Everyone is born as an "obligate nose breather," which means that people are programmed to breathe through the nose and not through the mouth. But in *every* single health fitness club across America that I've been in, I've noticed the vast majority of people have their mouths wide open.

Mouth breathing begins at an early age. People respond to stress by shifting into an emergency mode of breathing, but through the mouth simply because it's easier to do. Eventually, they start mouth breathing all the time.

When people breathe through the mouth they draw in a maximum quantity of air but fill only the middle and upper portions of their lungs. The blood supply needed for a quality exchange of gases (oxygen and CO_2) is found in the lower lobes of the lungs. For mouth breathing to supply enough oxygen to the blood, the body has to speed up breathing and heart rate. Such sharp rate increases make inefficient use of more oxygen and are believed actually to harm the system in some ways.

Nose breathing, on the other hand, engages the diaphragm, which then pulls air into the lower lung lobes first, where there is more blood available for oxygen exchange. And that takes the burden off the heart to pump faster. Among hunting-gathering societies, I've noticed that everyone engages in nose breathing. This way a vagal nerve stimulation is triggered that produces a calming, relaxed state for them. Aboriginal women are very laid back, slow, and easygoing individuals—quite a contrast, I must say, from their metropolitan counterparts in big-city America, who are generally wound tighter than clocks and run on nervous energy most of the time.

I've touched on the two most basic things that the average woman today needs to start implementing in her life if she expects to remain reasonably free of breast cancer. Thirty-minute walks a couple of times every day and nose breathing as you go along will help towards *reversing* some of those evolutionary biochemical body changes that are believed to be responsible for this terrible disease.

The Herb and Food Connection

The advice offered here is purely *nutritional,* nothing more than that. Publishers of alternative-health books tend to shy away from bold statements offering natural prescriptions for breast cancer. And since I'm not a licensed physician, I cannot legally or in good conscience dispense medical wisdom to deal with existing breast cancer.

But as a social scientist—a medical anthropologist—who has studied folk medicine worldwide for several decades, I can recommend some things that I *know* work for this type of problem. The mix of information will be helpful in both kinds of situations—to prevent breast cancer from occurring as well as to deal with existing cases of it.

From several hundred interviews in 19 years, conducted with women who've had breast cancer, I've discovered that two basic questions emerge: (1) "Will I die?" followed by (2) Will I lose my breast?" Confronting the reality of possible breast cancer is one of the most difficult things for a woman to do. It tends to send a shock through her female psyche and leaves a major psychological impact upon her system.

Therefore, certain *warm* herbal teas are usually suggested that will help to put her mind at ease and calm her wrecked nerves. Such brews include chamomile, peppermint, and couple of commercial blends that seem to work nicely for this. The two I have in mind are Women's Liberty and Nightly Night from Traditional Medicinals of Sebastopol, California. The former contains the woodsy taste of dong quai and angelica roots and the sweet and pungent flavors of licorice, ginger, cinnamon, and cloves. The latter is a nice blend of passion flower, chamomile, hops, spearmint, catnip, and other herbs to quiet the nervous system. All these teas are found in health food stores or herb shops.

The basic method for brewing such teas has already been given elsewhere in this book a number of times. But to repeat it here:

BREWING HERBAL TEA

Boil 1 pint of distilled or spring water. Add 2 tablespoons loose herbs or about 6 teabags. Gently stir, cover with a lid, and set aside. Steep for 20 minutes. Strain, if necessary, or remove teabags and drink 1–2 cups of *warm* tea on an empty stomach.

Next in line would seem to be those herbs that are either antibiotic in nature or that help to regulate hormone production in the body. The list below has been compiled over many years, from data gathered from alternative doctors and folk healers who routinely treat breast cancer patients.

Medicinal Plants	*Recommended Intake*
black currant oil	3 capsules daily with meals
borage oil	3 capsules daily with meals
echinacea	2 capsules twice daily without meals
evening primrose oil	3 capsules daily with meals
flaxseed oil (cold-pressed)	1 tbsp. daily with a meal
garlic (Kyolic with selenium)	2 capsules twice daily with meals
ginseng	1 cup tea daily
goldenseal root	2 capsules daily without meals (DO NOT take if you are hypoglycemic)
licorice root	1 capsule 3 times daily with meals
safflower OR sunflower oil	1 tsp. daily with a meal

Keep in mind that not all of these oils need to be taken at once. In fact, only a few from the recommended list are necessary at any given time. A woman may wish to choose one of these suggested options: black currant, echinacea, garlic, ginseng OR evening primrose, goldenseal, and safflower. In all cases, though, I would strongly advise taking licorice root with whatever selection options a woman chooses.

There is yet another herb with great therapeutic potential for women with breast cancer. In fact, this particular folk remedy has a lengthy history in American herbal medicine as being an outstanding agent against cancer. I'm speaking, of course, about red clover. It always seems to work better for this disease in the tea form than it does taken any other way. Follow the simple instructions previously given for Brewing Herbal Tea to make some of this for yourself. Drink up to 4 cups a day on an empty stomach for several months or as long as you deem necessary.

An imbalance in estrogen levels is thought by most medical doctors to be a triggering factor for many female-specific complaints: PMS, endometriosis, cervical dysplasia, or breast cancer. Substances containing isoflavones are believed to help normalize a woman's estrogen levels. To get more of these "hormone helpers" inside her body, a woman should eat more of these vital foods: soy products (tofu. soy milk, tempeh, miso), green peas, split peas, green beans, dried beans, lentils, garbanzos, and raw peanuts and peanut butter.

Juice Therapy Takes Over

Of all the things that have been mentioned in this section, I believe that certain juices form the best line of defense in a woman's body to help her resist getting (as well as treating existing) breast cancer. Some juices are already commercially prepared and easy for a woman to drink during her normal daily activities. I have in mind carrot juice (canned or bottled) or grape juice (usually bottled). A glass every day with or without meals is very handy to take. No preparation is required and minimal fuss is involved for a busy woman always on the go.

There are, however, a few other juices that need just a few minutes to make. But rest assured that they are well worth the time and effort put into them. To each recipe can be added the following *powdered* juice concentrates made by Pines International of Lawrence, Kansas (see Product Appendix for specific information).

JUICE CONCENTRATE POWDERS

1 tsp. Pines wheat grass

1 tsp. Pines barley grass

1 tsp. Pines organic beet root

$^1/_2$ tsp. Pines garden rhubarb root

Any of the foregoing amounts can be varied to suit individual taste preferences. But they greatly enhance the immune-boosting powers of several recipes listed here. NOTE: I suggest that a Vita-Mix Total Nutrition Center be used for making these juices, as it is the quickest and most efficient machine around for juicing purposes (see Product Appendix for details).

CITRUS POWER DRINK

$^1/_4$ pink or red grapefruit, peeled

$^1/_2$ orange, including white part of peel, quartered

$^1/_3$ cup pineapple, chilled

$^1/_2$ cup green or red seedless grapes

1 cup ice cubes

juice concentrate powders

Place all ingredients in the Vita-Mix container in the order given. Secure the lid and turn on the machine. Blend for $1^1/_2$ minutes until smooth. Makes $2^1/_2$ cups.

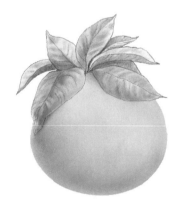

HOT MIXED-VEGETABLES TONIC

1 large tomato, quartered
$1/_4$ cup celery
15 sprigs parsley
1 tbsp. liquid Kyolic garlic
$1/_2$ green onion
$1/_4$ cup carrots
$3/_4$ cup water, boiling
juice concentrate powders

Place all ingredients in the Vita-Mix unit. Be sure the 2-part lid is tightly secured under both tabs so as no hot water will spill out causing an accidental scald. Turn the machine on and let it run for about $3^1/_2$ until smooth. Drink while still warm. Makes a little under 2 cups.

A woman should use juices whenever possible. They should be divided between *fresh* citrus fruits (for the vitamin C content) and *fresh* dark, leafy greens for the beta-carotene (vitamin A) present. These are really *the key* to breast cancer prevention and treatment.

BREAST CYSTS

Cleansing Teas to Flush Debris from a Woman's Body

DESCRIPTION

An estimated 37 percent of all women in America develop breast cysts between the ages of 33 and 52. As a rule, they are generally nothing to be concerned about. After the age of 30, glandular tissue in the breasts decrease and cysts form as a result of the normal aging processes.

Roughly 55 percent of those women who eventually develop breast cysts have only one, but a third of them go on to have multiple cysts, ranging anywhere from a pair to as many as five. Doctors find that the left breast is more likely to get a cyst than the right one. Cysts can either increase or decrease in size due to a variety of different circumstances.

Life and death on a cellular level are constantly going on within the body all the time. When the system is young, more new cells are being born there than are dying. But as the years set in, this ration is considerably reversed—old age implies nothing more than a larger abundance of cells ceasing to exist in proportion to a much smaller number being formed.

As with fallen leaves on the sidewalk or lawn in late autumn, so, too, does debris accumulate when a lot of cells finally die. This is essentially what forms the fluid found in a cyst. The color of it varies, of course, with the age of the cyst. The younger the cyst, the lighter in color and the thinner the fluid it contains, whereas in older ones, the color is much darker and the fluid a lot thicker.

Although not 100 percent certain, there have been enough medical studies published to suggest a strong link between multiple breast cysts and breast cancer. Therefore, it behooves a woman between the ages previously mentioned to do whatever she can to remove the cysts from her body.

The Miracle of Birch Bark Tea

Researchers at the University of Illinois in Chicago did something rather unusual in 1994. They went out and culled bark from a number of birch trees growing in a nearby parking lot. They took this material back to the laboratory and there extracted from the bark of the common white birch a naturally occurring substance called betulin. And from betulin they obtained betulinic acid and started testing it on human cancer cell cultures. They were amazed to find that tumor growths were "completely inhibited" by this stuff, while normal cells in the surrounding areas remained unaffected.

But something else just as good emerged when this extract of white birch bark was tested in animal models. When very high doses of betulinic acid were injected into mice, there were no manifestations of sudden weight change, diarrhea, or organ damage, which typically accompany nearly all anticancer drugs. The reports of this interesting piece of research, which appeared in the October 1995 issue of *Nature Medicine* and in the October 7, 1995, issue of *Science News* (148:231), both seemed to suggest that white birch bark was relatively safe for the human body.

This calls to mind an old Russian folk remedy I learned about during a visit I made to the Soviet Union some years ago in the company of a number of other scientists. The Russians had invested a lot of capital, time, and effort into the research of white birch. An elderly babushka (Russian grandmother) had shown some of them how she made a healing tea to treat breast cysts and breast cancer in a number of her female patients. These investigators followed her into the nearby woods and watched in silence as she methodically peeled off some of this bark in horizontal strips from white birch trees.

Everyone then returned to the old herbalist's house, where she proceeded to cut up the bark into smaller pieces using an old hatchet and heavy wooden block. Her host then boiled some water in a brass samovar (an urn with a spigot) before removing the top lid and throwing several handfuls of the bark inside. After replacing the lid, she let the mixture simmer for a while, then strained off the tea and gave each of the scientists who had come to watch these procedures a nice, hot cup of white birch tea.

Later on in their laboratories, these scientists were able to reproduce the same quality of tea, which they immediately tested on a number of volunteer women suffering from breast cysts or breast cancer. In 97 percent of the women who stayed with the tea for up to 5 months, virtually all of the cysts had disappeared. And in 67 percent of the women with cancer, who also drank the tea faithfully every day, where was a gradual reduction in the tumor size.

This information seems to suggest in a rather dynamic way that birch bark tea may be very useful as a detoxifying agent for the body in women suffering from either problem.

Other Blood Purifiers

There are many other herbs that work quite well in helping to rid the blood of many impurities. Some of these are readily available and quite affordable, while others are harder to find and tend to be more expensive. Two of my favorite herbs that appear to be effective in helping women get rid of accumulated dead-cell debris in their breasts are burdock and yellow dock roots.

It has been my experience that only the roots from the first-year burdock plants (those are the ones without the flower stalks) should ever be used. As is the character of biennials such as this, the first year is spent storing nutrition (often in the form of starch) in the thick root. But in the second year, the root becomes tough and woody because the plant expends all the stored energy in producing flowers and fruit.

On the other hand, the spindle-shaped yellow taproot of the second herb is best used in its second or third year, after it has had sufficient time to accumulate whatever iron and other minerals are present in the soil it grows in. There is also a rich, complex mixture of anthraquinones and anthraquinone glycosides, quite similar in nature to those found in cascara sagrada bark. It is these derivatives that produce the wonderful laxative effect characteristic of yellow dock root.

Both have been traditionally used to treat various skin diseases, benign skin tumors, knee joint swellings, fungal and bacterial infections, and liver problems. They work best as teas.

BIRCH BARK TEA

1/4 cup birch twigs

1/2 cup birch bark

3 cups distilled or spring water

Boil the water first. Then add the twigs and bark together. Cover with a lid and reduce heat. Simmer for 25 minutes. Set aside and steep for 10 minutes. Strain and drink 1 cup of *lukewarm* tea, flavored with honey or pure vanilla if necessary, on an empty stomach. Drink at least 1 cup each day for up to 5 months if needed. Store in the refrigerator for up to 3 days.

INTERNAL TEA RINSE FOR CLEAN BREASTS

3 tsp. burdock root

2 tsp. yellow root

3 1/2 cups <u>cold</u> distilled or spring water

Soak both herb roots in the cold water overnight. Next morning, bring the mixture to a boil. Set aside and steep for 15 minutes. Strain and drink one cup between meals every *other* day for 2 months. By then the cysts should be gone.

BREAST TENDERNESS

Things a Woman Can Do to Help Reduce Breast Hypersensitivity

DESCRIPTION

Breast tenderness can be due to a variety of things. Fluid-filled lumps induced by hormonal changes may cause breast thickening. A condition such as premenstrual syndrome can also contribute to the problem.

Doctors all too often are guilty of alarming women unnecessarily about breast tenderness. They still routinely diagnose the problem as fibrocystic breast disease, which is a term I think should be discarded from medical jargon altogether. It makes women think that their breasts are somehow diseased when, in reality, they're not. In fact, it's pretty normal for a woman's breasts to be just a little swollen sometimes.

Diet Change Is Necessary

Women with breast tenderness would do well to avoid caffeine and even decaffeinated beverages. It is believed by some doctors that compounds called methylxanthines, found in nonherbal teas, coffee, chocolate, and colas, may cause breast tenderness in some women. Something as innocuous as only *one* piece of chocolate during any given month can make some women's breasts hurt terribly.

Cream Rub and Oil Pack

Natural progesterone cream can help relieve breast tenderness. A woman should rub a little of it into the soft areas of her skin such as the inside of the forearms. This increases breast tenderness at first by temporarily increasing estrogen receptors in her breasts, but then the painful swelling gradually ebbs away and the breasts feel normal again.

Castor oil packs applied to the breasts three times a week for 45 minutes usually does the trick in doing away with breast tenderness. This treatment should go on for several months and then once a week thereafter.

GRANDMOTHER'S WONDERFUL TEA POULTICE

My aged grandmother Barbara Leibhardt Heinerman came from the old country of what was once Temesvara, Romania (but is now part of Hungary). She was an avid herbalist and practiced her craft in Europe and America with considerable dexterity and skill.

One of her best remedies that comes to mind for diminishing breast tenderness was a *cold* tea poultice. Here is how she made and applied it.

3 tbsp. grated <u>fresh</u> marshmallow root

1¹/₂ cups cold <u>seltzer</u> or mineral tonic water

Soak the root in the *cold* water overnight. *Do not boil!* Next morning, strain a small amount (maybe ¹/₂ cup) of the tea out into another cup. Take four cotton balls and work them together in pairs until you have only two larger cotton balls. Soak each of these in the tea, gently squeeze out excess liquid (but not too hard), and then place over each nipple and hold in place with Band-Aids or tape. If a larger area needs to be covered, make a double layer of gauze and cut out two circles about 2 inches in diameter. Soak each of them in the tea and apply the same way. Leave in place for an hour. Repeat several times throughout the day for up to a week if necessary.

BREECH BIRTH

Rapid Recovery from a C-Section for a New York Massage Therapist

DESCRIPTION

A birth this difficult is always manifested by the fetal buttocks being present in the maternal pelvis at the time of expected delivery. Breech delivery can be accomplished either vaginally or by Cesarean section (commonly called C-section). While it is possible for vaginal delivery, doctors usually prefer surgery, deeming it quicker and safer for both mother and infant.

Doctors Amazed by Quick Rebound

The following true story came to me entirely unsolicited from one Sharon Stolack of Westbury, New York. She is a 38-year-old massage therapist, who bought a copy of my best-seller, *Heinerman's Encyclopedia of Healing Juices.* She called me on the morning of Friday, October 6, 1995, to sing words of praise regarding what she felt was "a total health classic."

During our nearly hour-long conversation (on her nickel, of course), she related the following interesting experience. Sometime in 1992 she gave birth by C-section to a lovely daughter whom she and her husband named Shosana.

However, the surgeon who delivered the baby in this manner at Winthrop Hospital in Minneola, Nassau County, New York, was in for something of a shock. "He was astonished to see that I had *no fat* anywhere inside my intestinal tract, once he had cut me open," she said. "All of my epithelial tissue lining those cavities was orange-colored. He probably wondered what in the heck I had been eating or drinking to get this way," she said with a laugh.

What the doctor didn't know was that this patient of his was as healthy as a horse, on account of her vigorous lifestyle and very natural diet. Sharon had been drinking her own juice-and-syrup concoctions during much of her pregnancy. And as a result of this, she was up and around *in less than five hours!* Under normal circumstances, most women who have had a C-section require several days of bed rest before they can start walking very far again. Sharon was discharged in a matter of days as compared to a week for many other women in hospital maternity wards around the country.

SHARON'S REBOUND JUICE TONIC

12 oz. carrot

10 oz. beet

10 oz. cucumber

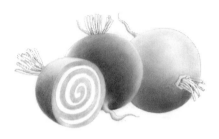

Juice all these together in advance; it makes a quart. Or put all of them into a Vita-Mix Total Nutrition Center in the order given, add 1 cup ice cubes, and mix for 2 minutes until smooth.

"I drank two quarts of this *daily* with one gallon of water," she stated. "And I fasted for three days in the hospital, never once touching any of their food. Instead, I opted to drink my juice tonic. I was out of there in *less* than three days, while every other mom in our C-section ward was there for at least a week!"

Staving off Anemia, Colds, Fevers, Fatigue, and Flus with Homemade Syrups

Sharon had some good health philosophy to share with America's women and wasn't at all bashful about telling me what she had on her mind. "Women need to know that the health food stores sell the *appearance* of health, but not always the *reality* of it. Sure, they go in and buy vitamin and mineral supplements by the cartload. But these things are merely *dried out* substances. They lack the electromagnetic energy that comes with juices. So instead of always popping health 'pills,' they ought to go out and buy juice machines and start juicing more. It would sure save them a lot of their hard-earned money," she said.

Well, this knowledgeable lady with the vibrant personality continued our lively discussion with more health tips for this book. She articulated everything so well that it made my job easier. Here is a recipe she makes with which to combat the common cold and influenza.

Sharon's Delightful Fig Syrup

1 gallon fresh spring water

2 cups cut figs (preferably the Turkish kind and unsulfured)

$1/_4$ tsp. garlic juice (or use 1 tsp. liquid Kyolic garlic in place of this)

Optional: 6 oz. celery juice; 6 oz. pear juice; 16 oz. green cabbage juice

Boil the water. Reduce to simmer. Add the figs and soak for 10 minutes. Set aside to cool. Then blend the water and figs together in a Vita-Mix Total Nutrition Center or equivalent food blender. Then add the garlic juice or liquid Kyolic aged garlic extract from Wakunaga of America (see Product Appendix for obtaining this).

Take 1 cup twice daily in between meals to keep up your immune system, Sharon stated. "It's the ultimate antibiotic to be taking when colds and flu go around," she thoughtfully observed. "One nice thing about it, though—you become an instant human insect repellent with the garlic!"

The other juices are optional and can be added in place of the garlic for different purposes:

celery juice for calming the nerves

pear juice for constipation

green cabbage juice for skin problems, flabbiness of skin, or constipation

Each of these items should be juiced alone and added *separately* to the fig syrup, but *not* all combined at once.

Sharon's Raisin Syrup

This one she uses for anemia, fevers, and fatigue.

1 gallon water

3 cups large ruby-red raisins

juice of 3 lemons

Follow instructions given in previous recipe. Drink one cup twice daily in between meals for wonderful rejuvenation. "There is no cure for anything," she concluded. "What we must do as women is to try and find ways to *perfect* our bodies."

BULIMIA

Answering Fear of Fat with Positive Nutritional Reinforcement

DESCRIPTION

Chamomile tea has a soothing effect on agitated nervous systems. And chlorophyll helps to strengthen the body when not much nourishment or anything else is getting onto the system, due to emotional or physical disturbances.

How Ellen Got Better

One of my former students, a 23-year-old college girl named Ellen, suffered from intense fear of becoming fat. She went through recurrent binge eating with periodic purging by self-induced vomiting, laxatives, and diuretics. A doctor knowledgeable about her malady diagnosed it as bulimia nervosa.

Ellen came to me for nutritional guidance. The fist thing I got her to do was finally to admit that she had a serious disorder. Second, she was encouraged to use some discipline and follow a self-supervised meal schedule. She was instructed to avoid bathrooms for at least three hours after each meal. She was told to monitor her weight every two days and to increase her physical activity.

Finally, I put her on a simple herbal program, consisting of a natural calming agent and a green food system intended for building some energy and stamina within her system. In a matter of weeks she had remarkably improved. Not only did she feel and look better, but her psychological state was more upbeat than it had been before.

MY SIMPLE PROGRAM FOR BULIMIA

STEP ONE

1 pint distilled water

2 tbsp. chamomile flowers

Boil the water. Add the herb. Stir and cover with lid. Set aside and steep for 15 minutes. Strain and drink one cup of *warm* tea 5 times a day.

STEP TWO

1 8-oz. glass spring water

**1¹/₂ tbsp. Pines Mighty Green health drink mix
(see product Appendix)**

Stir the Kyo-Green into the water thoroughly. Slowly *sip* the drink. Take several minutes until it is all gone. (*Do Not* hastily gulp it down!) Repeat this procedure at least three times a day in place of regular meals.

STEP THREE

Slowly begin introducing other *liquid* MEALS into the diet. They should be simple but tasteful. Hot soups and cool juices fit the bill best.

BURNS

A Religious Snake-Handler's Incredible Burn Remedy

DESCRIPTION

Burns are tissue injuries caused by application of heat, chemicals, electricity, or irradiation to the tissue. The extent of injury (or depth of the burn itself) is the result of the intensity of heat (or other exposure) and the duration of that exposure.

Burns are gauged in two different ways—partial or full thickness. First- and second-degree burns comprise the first category. The first-degree type involves superficial layers of epidermis. The second-degree kind involves varying degrees of epidermis (with blister formation) and part of the dermis. Third degree, however, is the only thing qualifying for full thickness; this involves the destruction of all skin elements with coagulation of subdermal plexus.

There are between 3 to $5^{1}/_{2}$ million estimated people burnt a year in America. A million or so of them require immediate medical care; there are an estimated 12,000 deaths annually from such unfortunate events. Burns are always the leading cause of accidental death in children.

Nothing to Fool Around With

While most *minor* burns can be effectively treated with alternative methods, readers need to use some common sense and realize that *serious burns deserve prompt medical attention* and should *not* be self-treated.

ElRoy's Onion Juice Poultice

There is a gentleman down Alabama way whom I interviewed awhile back with a mighty strange form of religious worship. He goes by the name of ElRoy and belongs to the Church of Jesus with Signs Following. Its members are mostly poor white Southerners, who take literally the biblical injunction that believers "shall take up serpents; and if they drink any deadly thing, it shall not hurt them."

Finding no place for themselves in modern industrial society, they've embraced a radical faith that allows them "the only power in

Christ Jesus that we have, as ElRoy explained to me. The Sacrament rituals here involve handling very poisonous snakes and guzzling strychnine to prove one's loyalty to the Master. "Christianity without a hint of danger to it, ain't fer much of a religion," ElRoy said with a toothless grin.

But I wasn't there to talk about whacky religious practices. Instead I had come to a part of rural Alabama to interview the man concerning his rather effective burn remedy, somewhat well-publicized in the region. I asked him how he had come about it, and he replied that his grandmother had developed it many years ago out of an emergency necessity.

ElRoy showed me how to make the remedy, which consists of turnip, onion, and olive oil. He took a medium-sized turnip and methodically grated it on a small hand-held metal grater until nothing remained of it but coarse pulp. This he put into a wooden bowl. Then he tackled the onion. To get juice out it, he first grated it while at the same time trying to fight off the tears due to the terrific sulfur fumes burning his eyes. The onion pulp was then put into the center of a square piece of muslin (about the size of an ordinary hanky); the corners were drawn together and the material was tightly twisted over the wooden bowl until about two tablespoonsful of juice had run out. One quarter of the onion pulp was added to the turnip matter and the rest dumped into a garbage pail. Finally, he measured out two teaspoonsful of extra-virgin olive oil and poured it into the bowl. He then mixed everything thoroughly with a wooden spoon.

"It's best not to use metal for putting this stuff in," he commented. "I like the wood myself, because I think it doesn't contaminate the remedy as much." The metal grater couldn't be helped, but is an essential tool to use in making the remedy.

Pretending that I had a second-degree burn on my forearm, he took me through the steps of his treatment. "First thing I tell 'em, is to remove all rings, watches, etc., from the injured area. Next comes off any clothing, and I cover the burned area with a dry sheet. Some injured folks are inclined to want me to put ice on their burns, but I tell them that only complicates matters more. Before I put this vegetable material on, I always lightly bathe the area with a strong solution of peppermint tea that I've had setting for a couple of hours around the cabin. It has a real cooling effect and helps to soothe the pain.

"I draw back the sheet each time the burn is to be treated. This way I know the injury won't get dirt in it." He then proceeded to apply his turnip-onion-juice-olive-oil mixture onto my arm with the short wooden spoon. Some of the stuff started falling off, so he stopped and loosely wrapped a thin layer of gauze around the arm to hold everything in place. "I keep it on for maybe about 12 hours before changing it again," he reckoned.

I've made only one modification to ElrRoy's grandmother's remedy. Knowing how vital it is that a burn victim consume a high-protein, high-calorie diet, I've added the following smoothie, for which I'm indebted to Bob Condor of the *Chicago Tribune* for sharing with me. It is his own humble creation of fruit juice and frozen fruit tailor-made for summertime sipping fun, but which I've found particularly useful for burn victims to drink. I've modified it just a bit by adding some protein.

Burn Smoothie for Fast Recovery

half a banana

$1/_2$ cup strawberries

$1/_4$ cup orange juice

$1 1/_2$ tbsp. of any good protein powder (this can be from soybean or a protein mixture used by some body builders for bulking up)

6 ice cubes

$1/_2$ cup milk (don't use 2%)

Combine everything in a food blender or Vita-Mix unit and mix for 2 minutes until a smooth consistency is achieved. Variations to this can be made by substituting other frozen fruits for the strawberries, or by substituting $1/_2$ to 1 cup of frozen vanilla yogurt for the ice cubes and milk. A little honey or molasses may be added if additional sweetening is desired. The burn victim should be given at least two of these every day, preferably about the same time that a new dressing is being put on.

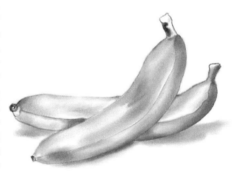

Other Benefits: Wounds and Fungal Infections Helped

At least one of ElRoy's three ingredients is very useful in treating wounds, sores, and fungal skin infections. A little bit of onion juice topically applied to these problems acts amazingly well in promoting more rapid healing of them.

Wrinkles Diminished

Still another ingredient of his remedy is very good for wrinkles. This is the olive oil, and while it won't necessarily remove wrinkles, it will help to diminish them somewhat. A little olive oil is applied to the area of each wrinkle. Then with the forefingers a gentle massage of the skin is commenced, going first in a clockwise circular motion, then back again counterclockwise. I had a French cosmetologist tell me this some years ago.

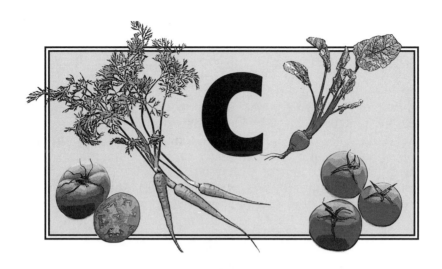

CANCER

The Late Ann Wigmore's "Answer to Cancer"

DESCRIPTION

Cancer has been with us, it seems, since the dawn of time. According to the scholarly treatise, *An X-Ray Atlas of the Royal Mummies* (Chicago: University of Chicago Press, 1980), some of the pharaohs of ancient Egypt were plagued with an odd assortment of different tumors. In modern times, cancer stands right behind heart disease and before strokes as being the second leading cause of death in our nation.

Those many individuals who are unfortunate enough to come down with some form of the disease usually are faced with considerable pain and misery, both physical and emotional, that always accompanies it. Its terrible effects on the human psyche and body are only compounded when the majority of its victims elect to go with medical science for treatments that can be as bad as the disease itself in most cases.

Marilyn Morris (her real name) is one such person who chose to go entirely the medical route. Her journey has been riddled with tremendous physical hurdles, unbelievable emotional potholes, and disastrous financial land mines. From September 29 to October 22, 1995, this 42-year-old mother of three underwent five surgeries, three standard chemotherapy treatments, and CAT scans of her head, chest, abdomen, and bones for advanced breast cancer and a harrowing bone-marrow transplant afterward.

She agreed to speak with members of the news media during and following her horrific ordeal. As an editor (five years) of Utah's largest, free-distributed newspaper *(Utah Prime Times)* for the senior community, I was able to garner some of the facts firsthand concerning her awful experience. When I saw her she had lost close to 20 pounds. And a visitor could have counted on both hands the few strands of hair remaining on her nearly bald scalp. She told me that she had been in and out of University Hospital in Salt Lake City almost two dozen times for a variety of blood tests and X-rays.

Without being disrespectful at all regarding the great suffering she went through, I couldn't help but think how much she reminded me of an alien lifeform from outer space the day I visited with her. There she was in her hospital bed with needles invading her veins and tubes snaking into her chest. Bone marrow had to be withdrawn from her hip (to be tested for cancer); this was quite an excruciating process, which she likened to "bumping down steel stairs on my ass."

Besides everything else, Marilyn had been injected with radioactive dye, infused with iodine, and forced to drink milky barium sulfate on numerous occasions, before spending endless hours under a room-size machine that explored the farthest reaches of her internal organs.

She groaned in obvious agony: "The diarrhea is terrible; I just wish I could get rid of it. And these horrendous stomach cramps are unbearable. My suffering is indescribable; it sometimes makes me wish I were dead already, but I intend to hang on to life as long as I can." Then after a moment's pause, she added reflectively: "Your body doesn't become your own. To my doctors, I'm just so much tissue without a personality."

Alternative Therapy that Is Low-Risk, Less Expensive, and Nearly Pain-Free

My heart went out to this poor woman. I so much wanted to tell her about some of the alternative treatment programs available to cancer victims that produce far less side-effects, are cheaper, more natural, and better for you. But how could I when she, her husband, her children, their extended families, and her many friends were 100 percent behind regular medical care for this frightening disease? How could I, as a minority of one, propose some very wonderful, but highly unorthodox remedies when I was heavily outnumbered and outvoted?

Therefore, I sadly but wisely passed that opportunity by and have decided to mention here in this book those things that I know work well for cancer, in the hopes that some of my readers may be more broad-minded in accepting health advice that the majority of doctors still view with considerable prejudice and tend to label as "medical quackery."

Meeting the Late Ann Wigmore: She Cured Herself of Colon Cancer at Age 50

The world lost one of its greatest advocates of healthy eating and natural living. Her name was Ann Wigmore, and she died from smoke inhalation in her Boston apartment on Thursday, February 17, 1994. She was 84 at the time of her untimely demise. Ms. Wigmore had been in the process of making some chamomile tea to help her sleep better, when the hot plate she was using for this suddenly caught fire.

I knew this grand dame of healthy living for more than a decade. We often met at various alternative-medical conventions where both of us were on the same program, but usually speaking at different sessions. We often spent quality time together comparing notes on different health-related matters. But it is probably fair to say that I learned more from listening to her than what I was probably able to teach her.

"Doctor Ann," as she was lovingly called by those who knew her well, never had any formal medical training. And she had little patience with scientists, believing them to be "dim-witted fools" which probably explains why I purposely kept my Ph.D. in medical anthropology in my back pocket and out of sight, once I learned her true feelings about college-educated people with degrees behind their names.

It was at the Health Horizons Expo held in Pittsburgh the weekend of November 4–6, 1983, at the old Soldiers and Sailors Memorial Hall on Fifth Avenue and Bigelow where she and I spent three to four hours discussing a wide range of health matters. It was probably one of the most meaningful interviews I've ever conducted in my life. Much of the information given here is from that interview and appears for *the first time* in print. Ironically enough, none of the holistic health journalists who had written about Ann through the years had ever probed as far into her personal life as I had. And she told me that by saying, matter-of-factly, "You're the first one I've ever let go this deep into my private affairs."

Ann Wigmore was born on March 4, 1909, on a farm in Cropos, Lithuania. She emigrated to America when she was 16 years of age. "I knew nothing about the laws of good health in those days," she sheepishly admitted. "My eating habits were very indiscriminate.

And I paid the price for it—by the time I was 50, my hair had turned completely white, and I suffered from arthritis, asthma, colon cancer, and migraine headaches. To have seen me then, you would have said 'there is one sick, old lady.' I was that far from the grave (holding a thumb and forefinger an inch apart)."

Desperate for help, Ann didn't know exactly where to turn. "At first I consulted with all the doctors, but soon found them to be a bunch of damned old fools who knew nothing and just kept people like myself in a constant state of sickness and pretty well doped up with drugs so we wouldn't feel so much of the pain."

Being of a religious turn—"I was born Catholic but switched to Methodist and Congregational"—she attended the Unity School of Christianity in Missouri. "This wasn't your typical theological school," she reminded me. "I received my ministerial license from them, but got my doctor of divinity from the College of Metaphysics." So, in the belief that the Universe had something more to offer her than did the "stupid philosophies of ignorant quacks" (meaning medical doctors), she turned to "the powers that be in the Great Beyond" (as she so eloquently phrased it). "I got the beginnings of my knowledge from the galaxy," she laughed. "Now how's that for believability?"

The "cosmic influences" from space (as she styled it), "told me that if I wanted to live, then I needed to stop eating 'dead food' and start eating 'living food.' It was plainly shown to me that 'living foods' had enzymes and vitamins in them. And that *fermented* foods were really good for the body because they were 'predigested,' that is to say partially digested, and therefore, could be more easily assimilated into the system with a minimum amount of digestive effort. *'These* are the foods,' I was told in plain English, 'that will destroy the cancers and other diseases in you and restore your body to good health again.' So, I became convinced then and there, to overhaul my life, get rid of all my old, bad habits, and begin anew with the things I'd been told to do."

Wigmore's "Answer to Cancer" Program: A Summary

"Dr. Ann's" natural approach to cancer involves a number of different elements. Some have to do with diet and herbs, while others focus more on lifestyle and psychological changes. They are each presented in detail under separate subheadings, but are briefly summarized here.

The first step involves preparing a simple, fermented wheat drink from wheat berries, which Ms. Wigmore referred to as Rejuvelac. The second calls for some rather creative and novel ways of using nuts and seeds. All three foods, she noted, provide a sick body with "predigested protein" to help it rebuild itself. The power of *fresh* juices came in third, but, in a sense, formed the nucleus of her outstanding nutrition program. For this reason there is more information on juicing than on any of the other steps involved.

The last two items she continually emphasized were a determined desire to get well and living in harmony with the environment around you. "I can't make people get well," she was always fond of saying. "I can only give them the *inspiration* for doing so. It is left for them to decide whether or not they really *want* to recover." And once recovery is evident, it is the duty of every former cancer patient to live in such an ordered way that everything between the body, mind, and spirit is in near perfect balance.

Rejuvelac, the "Miracle Food" for Getting Well

The first thing Ann started making was a simple, predigested food that she appropriately called Rejuvelac. She washed some whole grains of wheat enough times in a glass jar until the water ran clear. "I prefer organically grown wheat and the soft kind if it's available; but you can substitute the hard wheat, if necessary," she told me in our interview some years ago.

She then soaked one cup of wheat berries in three cups of water for 48 hours. The first soaking took her the longest time to ferment and would produce a mild-tasting Rejuvelac. "It's a good thing to have around the kitchen several stoneware crocks for fermenting and storing the finished drink," she added. She poured the first batch into an empty crock and used it as needed. The second batch was made by using the same seed from the first batch. Without rinsing the seeds, she added more water to the crock and permitted it to soak for just 24 hours. This batch, she assured me, wouldn't take nearly as long to ferment as it had already commenced fermenting.

Rejuvelac took the place of water and Ann started drinking it "by the quartsful." "This fermented wheatberry beverage of mine," she noted, "was the foundation on which I built everything else years later." Every sick person who walked into her ornate brick mansion, called the Hippocrates Health Institute, at the corner of Commonwealth Avenue and Exeter Street in Boston, and paid the standard $1,250 for a two-week stay received ample quantities of Rejuvelac. "It doesn't cure anything," she cautioned, "but only *builds the foundation* for the cure to rest on."

Predigested Protein from Seeds and Nuts

I can still remember that memorable visit we had with each other way back in 1983. Even after all these years, the humor, good-naturedness, and considerable health wisdom still shine through in that woman. In my heart I still feel an admiration for someone who fairly sparkled with humanity and compassion.

In that old Soldiers and Sailors Memorial Hall in downtown Pittsburgh, she continued spelling out for my benefit the details of her fascinating "Answer to Cancer" recovery program.

"The body always needs some form of protein," she said, "even when it's ailing and dying. I quickly discovered this with my own colon cancer—here I was wasting away into oblivion, but I couldn't eat any of the standard sources of protein, such as meat, milk, eggs, and butter. My body kept rejecting them."

So Ann ingeniously figured out her own "predigested protein," as she aptly named it. *"Everything* I consume is 'predigested!'" she stated with obvious enthusiasm. In other words, what she was telling me was that EVERY FOOD she consumed and gave to her many hundreds of patients to consume had in some way been FERMENTED! Her special "seed yogurt" became the *second* mainstay of her recovery program.

She experimented with different nuts and seeds to find out what each one tasted like. "Almonds are relatively sweet, sesame has a sharp taste, and sunflower seeds give a blander flavor," she observed. "Cashews are quite rich, but peanuts are difficult to digest. All the seeds become sweeter once they're sprouted."

To make her "seed yogurt," fill a two-quart glass Mason jar three-fourths full with seeds of your choice; they can be separate or mixed together. Figure on using 1 cup each of dehulled sunflower and sesame seeds. Pour over them $2^1/_2$ cups of Rejuvelac. Soak for $5^1/_2$ hours and sprout 13 hours. Blend with some more Rejuvelac (another $2^1/_2$ cups) to make a fine, thick cream. Pour this into a sprout bag made of muslin material and hang over a bowl to drip during the fermentation process.

"I always like to cut up some bell peppers, celery, and onions," she continued, "and mix them in with the seeds and liquid. When I add them I generally use a larger bowl to let everything ferment in. I keep it at room temperature the whole time it's fermenting. I cover the bowl, but never tightly. I let things sit for about five hours. Then I pour off the whey into another container. The seed yogurt can be refrigerated for several days. It has many uses. At the 'Mansion'

[Hippocrates Health Institute], we often add it to salads to make interesting creamy concoctions. I will even add a little bit sometimes to my green drinks, to give them more 'perk and spunk!' We use it just as we would yogurt, over fruit salads, as an in-between snack mixed with some Rejuvelac, and so forth.

"When I started putting this 'predigested protein' into my body, wonderful things began happening. My body experienced more energy, I gained weight, and my colon cancer started *diminishing!* No person with cancer should ever be without my Rejuvelac and this 'seed yogurt.'"

Juices Are the "Power of Life"

The late Paul Bragg had a very simple dietary philosophy that he lived by for most of his adult life: "Juices are the real *power of life,* and the more you consume them the longer you'll live!" He certainly was a living testament of this, dying in a drowning accident off Waikiki Beach, Hawaii, in December, 1976, just shy of his ninety-seventh birthday!

"Dr. Ann" also subscribed to the same ideology. "I could easily live to be 95 if I wanted to," I recall her telling me. At the time of our interview she described herself as "a feisty 75 year old" who was a "ball of energy." Dr. Bernard Jensen, a noted nutritionist, health practitioner, author, and speaker, still held to this "juicing theory" in the eighty-ninth year of his own existence.

Every one of these people were what might be called "apostles of good health and rightful living." Each one came from a troubled background filled with sickness, pain, and utter despair early in their lives. But the one thing they shared in common was that *fresh juices* helped them to fully recuperate and get their lives and health back in working order again.

Ann told me that after World War I there was "total devastation" of the area in which she and her family lived. So her grandmother Maria Warnisky went out with her and gathered "ordinary meadow grasses, like clover, lambsquarter, and timothy, and brought them home for us to eat," Ms. Wigmore recalled. "I never knew that such nourishing and simple meals could be made from *common weeds*. That experience helped to convince me later on in life that *grasses are essential* to making *worthwhile juices!* You just can't do without them. Practically no leafy vegetable can hold a candle to them in terms of the wonderful vitamin, mineral, and enzyme nourishment they provide."

Ann ranked the following plants as critical to cancer recovery and invariably included most if not all of them in her juices.

ALFALFA, because it is the "King of Mineral Content."

BEET, because its dark-red pigment enriches the blood.

CARROT, because it is high in antioxidant vitamin A components.

DANDELION, because it does the liver a world of good.

LAMBSQUARTER, because "wilderness nutrition" is at work here.

WATERCRESS, because of the valuable sulfur—a virtually unknown nutrient.

These six herbs, she felt, constituted "the perfect juice" for cancer prevention and treatment. While battling her own colon cancer, she not only drank two glasses of this mixture a day, but gave herself enemas with some of it, too.

Ann Wigmore's Juicing Secrets

I've modified some of "Dr. Ann's" recipe instructions to make it easier for readers to create it themselves. I also changed the name to reflect a broader, more positive use for this dynamic juice formula beyond its somewhat self-limiting and negative association with cancer. In fact, there are a number of other health benefits to it, some of which are cited near the end of this section.

JUICE POWERHOUSE

$1/2$ cup alfalfa sprouts

2 tbsp. Pines organic beet root juice powder (see Product Appendix for more information)

$1^1/2$ cups carrots, cut in 1-inch pieces

$1/2$ cup young dandelion greens

$1/2$ cup lambsquarter

$1/2$ cup watercress

2 cups water

2 cups ice cubes

1. Put the first three ingredients into a Vita-Mix container or equivalent food blender. Add 1 cup water and 1 cup ice cubes. Secure the two-part lid and run the machine for $1^1/2$ minutes.

2. Empty the contents into a large punch bowl or pot and set aside temporarily.

3. Put the container back on the machine (no need to rinse it out first).

4. Next add the remaining three ingredients and the other cups of water and ice cubes. Secure the lid and mix again for the same amount of time.

5. Empty these contents into the large bowl or pot and stir thoroughly with a wooden spoon.

6. Ladle equal amounts into two empty glass quart jars. Seal with lids and refrigerate. Drink one 6-fluid-ounce glass 4 times daily.

7. If some of it is intended to be used for an enema, make sure a little more water is added to dilute a bit, if necessary. Also, set it out several hours in advance so it reaches room temperature before injecting into the rectum.

The Urge to Get Well

The late Ms. Wigmore believed that discipline was critical to recovery. "While I may believe in compromising under certain circumstances," she once told me. "I've never done so when it comes to sick patients. Life has taught me that you can *never* compromise with illness. You must give a person sick with cancer or any other illness for that matter what he or she *needs,* and not what the individual may want. I don't pussyfoot around. Time is always of the essence when you have a serious, life-threatening disease on your hands. It is urgent that the person get back to health again as soon as possible.

"Four things I've found to be very helpful to me in treating sick patients. First of all, there must be a *desire* to heal and want to get well. Without it, neither the therapist in charge nor his patient under his immediate care will ever be successful in getting results that last. And once you and your patient have that desire, then both must *act upon it* while interest is still high and hope very strong. Also each one must *believe in it* or have faith that once the desire is acted upon it will eventually come to pass. The last thing is to always have *patience.* This is probably the one quality that so many therapists and patients lack. Nature works very slowly and the recovery process takes time, sometimes longer than we think."

Working in Harmony with Nature

Living in balance with your surrounding environment will keep you well in body, mind, and soul. One of Ann's statements culled from my lengthy interview with her back in the early winter of 1983 in Pittsburgh still stands out as being noteworthy and begs to be cited here.

"Sex is like food," she said. "If the person is upset, he or she will indulge in it or food or drink. That individual is always looking for a way out of the problem. But when the person is healthy and happy and productive, then he or she simply does not need overindulgence in anything, not in food, drink, or sex.

"If you teach an alcoholic restraint, he'll go off the sauce for a period, but then go right back on it again because the original cause for his drinking in the first place hasn't yet been removed. Or an overweight person, who is always stuffing his or her face with food. That person is doing so because there is a great deal of pain and sorrow there. But when someone is healthy, happy, and productive, then his or her expression comes from another direction. That's the way Nature works. Everything must sooner or later link up with Nature, because Nature always moves forward, is always evolving and growing.

"If we get linked up with Nature, then we automatically do what Nature does. I believe God and Nature are one and the same. And as we are one with Nature, so are we with God, too. But when we are not one with Nature, then we become abnormal in our behavior and habits. This lets disease in. Remember, though, that *nothing in Nature is ever abnormal!*"

Degenerative Diseases Show Improvement

Two components (Steps 1 and 3) of Ann's "Answer to Cancer" program are also of tremendous value in treating other problems. Degenerative diseases such as arthritis, diabetes, multiple sclerosis, and systemic lupus erythematosus respond very well to Rejuvelac and Juice Powerhouse. Three cups of the former and one of the latter each day with meals will help turn around any of these conditions.

CANDIDIASIS

(see Vaginitis and Yeast Infection)

CATARACTS

Nutritional Support for More Clear Vision

DESCRIPTION

Cataracts are a common eye condition in many people over the age of 65. This occurs when the eye lens is unable to correctly focus upon objects near or far away, due to a cloudy or opaque situation.

Suggested Supplements

In addition to Rejuvelac (previously mentioned under CANCER), sprouts, and mixed greens/carrot juice combo recommended by the late Ann Wigmore, certain health food supplements will also be of definite benefit. Vitamin A intake should not exceed 50,000 I.U. per day; this should be divided between fish oil (25,000 I.U.) and beta-carotene (25,000 I.U. also). About 2,000 mg. of nonacidic vitamin C, in evenly divided doses morning and night, is advisable. Vitamin E intake should never exceed 600 I.U. daily; wheat germ oil is a good source for this. A high-potency B-complex vitamin (3 tablets daily) is, likewise, recommended. Finally, a fluid extract of bilberry (30 drops orally) is essential to improving failing vision.

CAVITIES

Green Tea High in Natural Fluoride, Which Prevents Tooth Decay

DESCRIPTION

Tea is still the number one drink in the United Kingdom. The prestigious British Tea Council estimates that approximately four cups of tea per person per day is drunk in Great Britain alone. The Brits drink two and a quarter cups of tea to every cup of coffee, and four cups of tea to every equivalent unit of soft drink. In the early 1990s the United Kingdom roughly consumed a fifth of the world's tea production.

The British custom of afternoon tea was originated about 1840 by the Duchess of Bedford. Iced tea was introduced at the St. Louis World's Fair of 1904 by Richard Blechynden, an Englishman who, unable to sell the heated beverage because of hot weather, poured it over ice.

Tea is commonly sold in loose form, in filter-paper tea bags, or in soluble form. Tea bags were introduced by Thomas Sullivan, a New York wholesaler who sent tea samples to his customers in small silk bags instead of the usual tins. Instant teas, first produced in the 1940s, include flavored and cold-water-soluble types.

The majority of Britons prefer taking their tea with a little bit of milk in it. This is similar to many Americans liking their coffee with a small amount of cream added.

Dentists Encourage Tea Drinking to Prevent Caries

Within the last decade tea drinking has received a big boost from some of America's dentists. In an article, "Drink Tea, America," which was published in the journal *Dentistry 86* (April 1986, pp. 20–21), the following conclusions were arrived at:

> Some natural foods are good for oral health because of constituents that interfere with bacterial colonization and subsequent acid formation. Commercial drinking tea . . . is a cut above other beverages in its natural anticariogenic properties. . . . Tannins and fluoride give tea a unique anticariogenic potential without undesirable side effects.

Fluoride is believed to be one of the compounds responsible for this remarkable anticariogenic activity. Dentists routinely use fluoride in their practice. Many large metropolitan water supplies are fluoridated to help reduce the incidence of tooth decay in children. And a large number of commercial toothpastes have fluoride in them as well.

Those who oppose synthetic fluoridation for personal health or ethical reasons will be happy to know that green tea contains *twice* as much *natural* fluoride as does black tea. According to the *Chinese Medical Journal* (24:55–61, 1977) green tea automatically has the highest amount of natural fluoride because it has *not* been fermented. Black tea, on the other hand, which has been fermented for the longest time, has the lowest amount of this important trace element. "The anticariogenic effect of teas . . . decreases proportionally to the degree of fermentation," the article noted.

Research Shows "Why" Tea Prevents Cavities

"Every time you eat a sweet," Isao Kubo's grandmother used to say, "drink some green tea." Though Kubo failed to heed her advice and ended up with a mouthful of cavities (for which he needed plenty of dental work done), he now acknowledges that he should have. An organic chemist, Kubo reported data to the American Chemical Society's spring meeting in San Francisco in April, 1992, that demonstrated that flavor compounds in Japanese green tea can kill *Streptococcus mutans*—bacteria that help initiate dental caries.

The tea's cavity-fighting potential, confirmed roughly a decade before this, first seemed to be connected to water-soluble compounds, largely tannins, that can halt *S. mutan's* production of glucans. These sticky materials bind acid-generating bacteria to teeth. But a cup of tea didn't appear to contain enough glucan inhibitors to account for its anticariogenic activity. So Kubo turned to green tea's hexanes—oily, floral-scented, water-insoluble compounds that give the drink its distinctive flavor.

At least nine of the ten most abundant flavor compounds in green tea also inhibit glucan production, Kubo's team of researchers at the University of California, Berkeley, reported. Moreover, when certain of these hexanes accompany one another, as they do in the tea, they can kill the microbes—and at far lower levels than required to shut down glucan production.

But an interesting social problem arises: What if you happen to be Mormon or Seventh-Day Adventist and aren't supposed to be drinking green or black teas on account of their caffeine contents? Being a Latter-Day Saint myself, I posed this question to Dr. Kubo. He responded by telling me that these same active hexanes found in green tea also occur naturally in coriander, sage, and thyme. "If your religion doesn't prohibit them," he finished, "then I would suggest making a tea out of any of these and rinsing your mouth after every meal."

Green Tea Preparation

Orientals prepare their tea a lot differently from the way the English or Americans do. For one thing they don't steep it as long, and, for another, tea drinking in the Orient has become a ritual ceremony in many places. Elsewhere in this book I've given other instructions on how to prepare tea that will be somewhat different from what is mentioned here. The apparent contradictions are easily resolved once you understand that for purposes of cavity prevention, the tea doesn't need to be steeped for very long. In fact, the *least* amount of time that green tea for rinsing the mouth and teeth after a meal is exposed to heat is preferable.

The standard method goes something like this: Combine one rounded teaspoon of any type of green tea in water that has *cooled slightly* after boiling; steep it for *no more* than $1^1/_2$ minutes before rinsing and gargling with it.

CELLULITE

A Proven Remedy for a Distressing Women's Problem

DESCRIPTION

Some two decades ago (1975) a best-selling book dealing with a presumed condition that was termed *cellulite* hit bookstores nationwide. That's when the word was first coined, and a few million women started having angst about the dimpling effects in their fannies and thighs. Ever since then desperate females of all ages, wanting to have firm thighs and toned buttocks, have wasted hundreds of millions of dollars on products and treatments promising to get rid of such bumpy lumps of fat.

But, in all honesty ladies, cellulite is *not* a disease. Heck, it's not even abnormal, for that matter. It just *is* there on your bodies, because of the way your gender packs its excess fat around. The dimpling is produced by fibrous cords that connect the skin to underlying muscle tissue in the thighs and buttocks. These cords tether the skin to the deeper structures, with the fat lying between the layers. As fat cells accumulate, they push up against the skin, bulging around the long, tough cords.

What's even more ironic is that you won't find the term mentioned in most medical books dealing with human anatomy. The closest reference I came to it in *Stedman's Medical Dictionary* (25th Edition) (Baltimore: Williams & Wilkins, 1990, p. 273) listed it simply as a conversational word "for deposits of fat and other material *believed* (read: "imagined") to be trapped in pockets beneath the skin."

What Really Works for Getting Rid of Ugly Cellulite

Okay, so I've proven to you that, technically from a medical and scientific perspective, the condition simply doesn't exist. That may be all fine, well, and good for myself as an anthropologist to declare, but for you, dear readers who are women with cottage-cheese thighs and behinds there is little comfort to be found in the facts just presented.

So, I'm going to switch from technical explanations and give you a remedy that I know works *fairly* well for helping to get rid of *some* of your cellulite. But please give a moment of your attention to the previously italicized words—the words "fairly" and "some" give real clues as to just how effective this remedy really is and how much cellulite you can honestly expect to lose.

My secret weapon in the war against cellulite comes from the Orient. *It is green tea.* I had wondered for years, while traveling throughout Southeast Asia, why *so few* Chinese, Japanese, Korean, Thai, and Indonesian women were ever bothered with cellulite. I posed this to more than one Oriental doctor I met in my numerous travels to these parts of the world. And always the same answer kept coming back to me, expressed in different ways: "Our women drink green tea all the time, but your American women do not."

While I've obviously given you the key now to getting rid of some of your cellulite, what I can't tell you is exactly how much to take or for how long. You see, that is an individual thing, based entirely upon your own body chemistry, age, height, and weight. One woman reading these words, who may be thirtysomething, weighs 135, is 5'11" tall, and has normal hormone production might be able to drink two cups of green tea a day and have 80 percent of her cellulite gone within a matter of *months.* On the other hand, another female reader who happens to be in her menopause years, tips the scales at 180+, stands in stocking feet at 5'2" high, and has a yo-yo kind of hormonal makeup could be drinking five cups a day for six months and realize only a modest decrease of 20 percent reduction in her overall body cellulite content.

You will just have to experiment a little before determining how many cups of tea a day and for how long would be right for your body. A little hint, however: *Daily* exercise in the form of *walking* for 30 minutes, immediately *following* ingestion of *two* cups of green tea, has been known to modestly accelerate cellulite reduction. Good luck in your efforts.

CERVICAL CANCER

Juice and Tea Douches as Useful Adjuncts to Regular Medical Treatment

DESCRIPTION

A woman's cervix is located at the end of her vaginal canal, marking the entrance to her uterus. It is the most common site of gynecological cancer. Cervical cancer is the growth of malignant cells in this narrow opening of the uterus. Cervical cancer develops slowly from a distinct precancerous stage (called dysplasia). Cancer can either be confined to the surface (preinvasive) or else spread more deeply into the cervix or other organs (invasive).

Lifestyle Changes to Reduce Your Risks of Getting It

As more and more people turn to food supplements for improving their overall health, there is a false assumption in the minds of many that if they take adequate amounts of vitamins A (50,000 I.U.), C (3,000 mg.), and E (400 I.U.) every day, watch their diet, and control their stress, that this will prevent them from ever getting cancer. Admittedly, all of these things are important, but they form only *part* of the picture.

Changing certain lifestyle *habits* is the other missing 50 percent. Girls and young women should avoid having sex at too early an age. There should *never* be multiple sexual partners, just *one*. Synthetic hormones like DES should *not* be taken during pregnancy. And women who smoke, *shouldn't!*

All of the foregoing suggestions were arrived at by myself over a period of many years studying numerous women in many Third World countries who are absent of cervical cancer. The things I cited are *not* moralistic pronouncements by me. Instead, they are a compilation of things I observed with the women I was around in other nations. Take these things for what they're worth and govern yourself accordingly.

Douching with Juices and Teas

Women who have cervical cancer in various stages of development and are looking to this book for alternative solutions to their problems must understand one thing—*I am not a medical doctor.* I don't profess to treat patients. What I am, though, is a medical anthropologist who studies folk remedies worldwide and then applies the best of them in self-care health books such as this one. I am of the opinion that in situations such as cancer, a person ought to borrow from *both* systems of medicine, the orthodox as well as the alternative, and form a treatment program that suits him or her best.

Red clover tea is an excellent thing to be taking internally if you have cervical cancer. I recommend 3 cups a day, between meals. Chaparral tea is good for douching; I suggest $1^1/_2$ cups twice each day for this. Carrot juice is good for you on account of its high beta-carotene content; try drinking at least 2 cups a day with meals. A liquid chlorophyll-garlic is handy for douching; $^3/_4$ cup twice daily is recommended. The same amount should also be taken orally. One level teaspoon of liquid Kyolic garlic from Wakunaga (see Product Appendix) will replace the juice of raw garlic.

Effective Douching

Douches have been with women almost since the time of Mother Eve. Appliances that have been used for this purpose include a water bottle with hose attachment, a small bulbous syringe (similar to what is used for giving an infant an enema), and, of course, the standard douche bag. When douching with any of the aforementioned teas or juices, I would recommend that they be *slightly* diluted with this combination medium: 1 tablespoon of apple cider vinegar, 1 teaspoon of 3 percent hydrogen peroxide, and one pint of spring or distilled water.

When taking a douche, the tip of the appliance to be used should be carefully inserted and the vaginal opening well-sealed with the hand so the fluids can fill, stretch, and cleanse all parts of the vagina. A woman with cervical cancer should try to retain the liquid contents as long as possible, before her body wants to have them expelled. Douching like this twice or three times daily is helpful in reducing the cancer, but not necessarily in getting rid of it. A strict diet, ample vitamin-mineral supplements, and antibiotic herbs such as echinacea, Kyolic garlic, goldenseal, and pau d'arco are, likewise, required for additional support. The first three herbs can be taken in capsules (about 4 a day of each), while the last one works best in fluid extract (20 drops under the tongue twice daily).

MAKING HERBAL TEA DOUCHES

Boil 1 pint of water. For red clover tea, add 2^1/$_2$ tablespoons of dried blossoms. Cover, set aside, and steep 20 minutes. Strain and use as previously directed. For chaparral tea, add 2 tablespoons of dried plant material. Cover and simmer on low heat for 20 minutes. Set aside and steep overnight for 8 to 10 hours. Strain and use as formerly instructed. NOTE: *Teas to be injected into the vagina should be room temperature and never cold!*

MAKING HEALING JUICES

A nifty carrot juice recipe courtesy of the Home Economics Department of the Vita-Mix Company is easy to make and delicious to drink. I've modified it slightly.

> *1 cup goat's milk, room temperature*
>
> *1 cup carrots (preferably organic)*
>
> *^{1}/$_2$ cup apple juice (canned or bottled), room temperature*

Place all ingredients in a Vita-Mix Total Nutrition Center container and lock the two-part lid in place. Turn unit on and permit it to run almost two minutes. Drink several cups daily with food.

The chlorophyll-garlic combination intended for douching is even simpler than the former to make.

> *1 cup warm water (spring or distilled)*
>
> *1 level tsp. Mighty Greens Health Drink Mix*
>
> *1 tsp. liquid Kyolic garlic*

Stir everything thoroughly together by hand or else blend in a Vita-Mix unit and use as previously directed. NOTE: Remember to *dilute* slightly with the previously suggested items.

CERVICAL DYSPLASIA
Food Helps for Abnormal Pap Smears

DESCRIPTION

Cervical dysplasia is what doctors call any abnormal cellular activities going on deep within the cervix itself. Unless a doctor is sensitive to a woman's emotions, he or she is apt to unwittingly induce panic in the female patient by casually announcing that her Pap smear was abnormal, without additional qualifying comments. A woman should know that just because her Pap smear came back abnormal *doesn't* mean she is a candidate for cervical cancer; in fact, most cases of cervical dysplasia *never* develop into cancer.

Scientific research has determined that *how* a woman functions mentally and emotionally will usually indicate the mildness or severity of her cervical dysplasia. A woman who lets others dominate her, has low self-esteem, and is pessimistic about things in general often has severe cervical dysplasia. On the other hand, a woman who is strong-willed, independent, and upbeat about life usually has a mild case.

Food Therapy that Works

The key to treating this problem nutritionally is to consume foods rich in vitamins A and B-complex and folic acid (one of the B vitamins). Carrots, kale, spinach, and sweet potato are all high in vitamin A. Food sources rich in folic acid/folacin include desiccated liver (available at most health food stores) and species of lettuce (bib, Boston, romaine). A high-potency B-complex vitamin (2 tablets daily) is also recommended for this problem.

A Testimony of Juicing

Irene W. of Hackensack, New Jersey, told me the following true story some time ago.

> "I went to my doctor to have the usual Pap smear. He used a soft brush [called a cytobrush] to take a good sample of cells up inside my cervical opening. He then fixed these cells onto a glass slide by spraying them with some kind of cell-preserving chemical. He had a member of his staff trained to read cellular abnormalities, examine them beneath a microscope.
>
> "My doctor came back and told me that my Pap smear indicated that I had an SIL 4, which is considered pretty severe. I damn near panicked and thought I had cancer on the spot!" (*NOTE:* SIL is the

112

medical abbreviation for squamous intraepithelial lesions, which signifies that abnormal cells are in the squamous layer covering the cervix, vagina, or vulva. SIL is slowly replacing an older term CIN, which stands for cervical intraepithelial neoplasia.)

"Well, I followed the advice you gave me over the telephone and started juicing. I bought a Vita-Mix machine like you suggested and followed your instructions to the letter. I went back some six weeks later and had not only another Pap smear but also a cervigram." (*Note:* A cervigram is a photograph taken by the doctor of the cervix at the same time he or she administers the Pap smear.)

"The medical report came back that both tests were negative. The doctor was astonished that my cervix was now 90 percent normal again. He couldn't believe how this reversal had happened so quickly. Thank you for your help."

THE VEGETABLE JUICE COMBO IRENE USED

2 cups spring or mineral water (cool)

$^3/_4$ cup carrots, cut in 1-inch pieces

$^1/_2$ cup kale

$^1/_2$ cup spinach leaves, snipped into small pieces

$^1/_4$ cup <u>cooked</u> sweet potato (peeled)

1 tsp. Pines Mighty Greens health drink mix

1 tbsp. liquid Kyolic Garlic from Wakunaga

$^1/_2$ tsp. desiccated liver powder

1 cup ice cubes

Place all ingredients in a blender container or a Vita-Mix unit in the order given. Secure the lid and blend on HIGH speed for 2 minutes until smooth. Makes about 2 cups. Drink with a meal.

CERVICITIS

(see Vaginitis)

CHILDBIRTH PAIN

(see Labor)

CHOLESTEROL (ELEVATED)

(see Obesity)

CHRONIC FATIGUE SYNDROME

Marketing Manager's Great Love Affair with Herbal Tea Blends

DESCRIPTION

Chronic fatigue syndrome (CFS) is characterized primarily by profound fatigue, in association with multiple systemic and neuropsychiatric symptoms lasting at least six months and often severe enough to reduce or impair daily activity. It affects the endocrine/metabolic and musculoskeletal systems. An estimated 7.5 million Americans are afflicted with it, most of them young adults and the greater majority of them female. Herewith is a laundry list of typical signs and symptoms with percentages of how often they appear:

fatigue (100%)

ability to date onset of illness (100%)

unexplained general muscle weakness (90%)

joint pain (90%)

forgetfulness (90%)

inability to concentrate (90%)

emotional instability (90%)

muscle pain (90%)

confusion (90%)

mood swings (90%)

low-grade fever (85%)

irritability (85%)

prolonged fatigue lasting 24 hours after exercise (80%)

depression (80%)

headaches (76%)

abnormal visual intolerance of light (76%)

difficulty sleeping (76%)

allergies (70%)

vertigo (40%)

enlargement of the lymph glands (40%)

shortness of breath (33%)

chest pain (33%)

nausea (33%)

weight loss (30%)

hot flushes (30%)

irregular heart beats (30%)

excessive tenderness and pain in lymph nodes (30%)

discomforts in the G.I. (gastrointestinal) tract (30%)

night sweats (25%)

unexpected weight gain (not due to pregnancy) (15%)

unexplained rash (15%)

The foregoing data were obtained from statistical information supplied by epidemiologists working at the Centers for Disease Control in Atlanta, Georgia.

Romancing the Teas

Robin Eberhardt is a vivacious and energetic 29-year-old married woman who is part of the winning team responsible for the production and distribution of all my health best-sellers put out by my publisher, Prentice Hall of Englewood Cliffs, New Jersey. She has been romancing a number of herbal tea blends now for quite some time to correct occasional energy deficiency problems.

"My great love affair with teas," she began her letter to me, "started at a restaurant on my first business trip after graduating from college eight years ago. I asked for tea, and the waiter presented me with a cherry-wood box filled with different types of tea. This overwhelmed me at the time, since I knew only of basic Lipton orange pekoe and pekoe cut black tea. Since then I have broadened my selection to include all types of herb and fruit teas.

"In the morning I enjoy drinking teas that rejuvenate me and make me feel alive and ready to tackle all the challenges ahead. Some of my favorites include: Celestial Seasonings "zinger" teas such as wildberry zinger, lemon zinger, blackberry zinger, and orange-mango zinger. I find the natural fruity taste to be quite zesty and peppy, not to mention light, since tea contains zero calories.

"In the evening when I want to relax and unwind from a stressful, busy day at work, I drink Lipton Soothing Moments teas, in particular, their golden honey lemon and country cranberry. Sleepytime Cozy Chamomile tea is also quite soothing. These teas also help lift my spirits when I'm 'blue' or depressed in spirits. Peppermint tea is wonderful for an upset stomach.

"Celestial Seasonings Country Peach Passion tea and strawberry kiwi tea make for a nice sweet treat. Both have a tropical twist and are quite luscious. The fruit flavor and fragrant smell really do the trick for me."

I couldn't help noticing her reference to these particular teas as being "a nice sweet treat." A common trait shared by those who suffer from chronic fatigue syndrome or hypoglycemia is that both groups have an irresistible craving for sweets. And whenever they indulge themselves in sugary foods there inevitably follows severe drops in body energy levels a short time later. So, what seems to make sense here is that teas with fruity aromas and flavors to them be used frequently by those who like sweets a lot in order to at least satisfy the mental cravings for sugar.

She concluded her memo by noting: "It's very easy for me to 'escape' from life for a moment while drinking these teas. Just holding a warm filled mug changes my focus and either calms or rejuvenates me." Stress is bad for anyone, but especially for those with chronic fatigue or low blood sugar. And the stress imposed upon such bodies by inclement, cold weather can be murder on their systems. I've had many people with either or both problems tell me time and again that it felt as if they were "dying inside" during the winter and actually dreaded the arrival of the cold temperature season. Warm teas, such as those Robin enjoys, will help alleviate some of the stresses that winter puts on those with chronic fatigue or hypoglycemia.

Nutritional Support for Chronic Fatigue

Ms. Eberhardt's pattern of eating is also interesting in light of each disorder being discussed here. Doctors often advise their patients with fatigue and blood sugar problems to "eat more frequently throughout the day" instead of just the three standard square meals that most of us are used to. This way constant fuel is being supplied to the body, so that energy reserves don't run low. Robin described herself as "more of a grazer," tending to "eat something every couple of hours or in small bits." She's a big fan of grains (cereals, breads, and pretzels) and pastas, but also loves fruits, vegetables, yogurt, beef, and chicken. She eats "desserts sparingly." The only part of her diet that doesn't fit at all to help chronic fatigue or hypoglycemia sufferers is the consumption of fruit (or fruit juices) and desserts—they should be *avoided* under such circumstances.

Robin takes different nutritional supplements to help maintain her healthful and very active lifestyle. I was surprised by the fact that some of them were also recommended for both problems. (See James F. Balch, M.D., *Prescription for Nutritional Healing* (Garden City Park, NY: Avery Publishing, Inc., 1990; pp. 136, 212). Her daily program includes the following nutritional supplements:

a multivitamin—3 capsules
vitamin A—25,000 I.U.
vitamin B-complex—100 mg.
vitamin C with bioflavonoids—500 mg.
vitamin E—400 I.U.
calcium-magnesium—1,500 mg.
selenium—200 mcg.

Other nutrients not taken by her but very helpful for chronic fatigue syndrome and hypoglycemia include:

a multimineral—2 capsules
Kyolic EPA (aged garlic extract)—2 capsules
Ginkgo Biloba Plus from nakunaga—2 capsules
iron—18 mg. (should always be taken separately)
chromium (GTF)—100 mcg.
kelp (for the iodine content)—3 capsules
yarrow herb (for painful inflammation)—4 capsules
zinc—50 mg.
Kyo-dophilus—1 capsule
amino acid complex—use as directed on label
Pines Mighty Greens drink mix—1 tablespoon in 8 fl. oz. water

All of the above can be found in your local health food store. The Kyolic EPA, Ginkgo Biloba Plus, and Kyo Dophilus are all manufactured are all manufactured by Wakunaga of America (see Product Appendix for additional information on them).

Energy-draining problems such as chronic fatigue syndrome, hypoglycemia, and candidiasis (yeast infection) are discussed in much greater detail in another book of mine, *Double the Power of Your Immune System* (Englewood Cliffs, NJ: Prentice Hall, 1991). Pages 24–35, 223–228, 297–301, and 302–304 are especially helpful in the information they provide. Interested readers are encouraged to contact the publisher for copies of this definitive work by calling 1-800-947-7700.

Keeping Busy Distracts Attention

One final thing I believe needs mentioning here is Ms. Eberhardt's *enriched* lifestyle. This assistant marketing manager, whose many duties at Prentice Hall include handling the huge mailings for all my books, occupies herself in pursuits that are fulfilling and quite satisfying. These include walking, occasional light aerobics, reading (she likes John Grisham novels and business and self-improvement books), music (jazz, contemporary, and alternative or New Wave rock), volunteer work (American Cancer Society), and many small "day trips" (street fairs, balloon festivals). Although not a homebody in the traditional sense, she is still very family-oriented (spends time with her nieces) and enjoys pets very much ("I have an interest in cats").

The point to be made here isn't so much to reveal to the world what this vibrant personality does with her private life, but rather to show that *she keeps herself busy* with things she likes. I've noticed that many people who suffer from chronic fatigue or hypoglycemia nearly always seem to feel sorry for themselves. Maybe they're so preoccupied with their own health problems that they fail to smell the flowers, hear the warbling of songbirds in the treetops, feel the breeze or gentle wind, and, in general, take better notice of the wonderful world around them. This is what Robin Eberhardt has managed to do, and I think that her activities in these things makes a fine example for the sick, tired, and ill-humored to follow for brightening up their own lives more.

Other Benefits: Recuperation from Illness or Surgery

Herbal teas are certainly ideal to use for those just recovering from a recent illness or surgery. Such teas invigorate the body and enliven the senses; they create a more hopeful mood and a better outlook on life. Any of the teas previously suggested by Ms. Eberhardt would be helpful in such instances.

Rinsing the Body of Debris

Just as one might take a garden hose with attached nozzle, turn on the water pressure, and wash down the sidewalk and driveway of one's house, so too do teas work in a similar fashion inside the body. They help to get rid of accumulated debris from some of the junk we eat and drink, and they flush harmful chemicals and bacteria from our bodies. We tend to feel a lot better after drinking herbal teas of our choice.

COLITIS

State Trooper Helped with Papaya Juice and Chamomile Tea

DESCRIPTION

Having been to Panama several times on research expeditions for more folk medicine remedies, I learned a lot about papaya that I never knew before. Let me share some of these things with you now.

The Ailigandi Cuna down there apply the caustic latex yielded by the unripe fruit to infected sores; one application is all that's necessary to clear things up. The pith of the young papaya stems sometimes serve as famine food during periods of extreme food shortage.

Many Panamanians use the papaya leaves to tenderize meat. Natives frequently wrap meat overnight in the leaves and then cook it in the same leaves the next day. Sometimes a little of the blistering milky juice is dropped into the cooking pot before tough meat is added. Meat tenderized this way often develops a peculiar flavor. Some residents in that Latin American country informed me that animals fed papaya seeds before being slaughtered had more tender meat.

Papaya leaves are employed in washing clothes. The pulp of ripe papaya fruit is frequently used in shampoos and face creams. The latex is often used to remove warts, freckles, and other blemishes.

A number of Panamanians I interviewed also rely on chamomile (manzanilla in their language) to help relax their nerves, give them a good night's sleep, and settle upset stomachs. They take it as a warm tea with or without meals.

"But Officer, I Wasn't Going THAT Fast . . . Was I?"

We're actually dealing with *two* distinct problems here—one that is health-related and the other that is traffic-related. May I advise you in advance that if you're planning to drive through the Beehive State anytime soon on I-15 South, that you be on the lookout for Lt. Jones, an eager beaver with the Utah Highway Patrol who just l-o-v-e-s to fill up ticket books by the dozens with the names of all those drivers suffering from "lead-foot syndrome."

Officer Jones and I met the usual way: I was doing 90 in a 65-mile-an-hour zone and he was intent on ticketing me for breaking the law.

119

"What's your hurry, Dr. Heinerman?" he politely inquired after checking over my license and vehicle registration.

"I'm on my way to the Las Vegas Convention Center to autograph about 500 copies of one of my many health books. It is entitled *From Pharaohs to Pharmacists: The Healing Benefits of Garlic* (New Canaan, CT: Keats Publishing, Inc., 1994; 196 pages).

"Oh, so you write books about herbs and stuff like that?" came the rhetorical question. "Yeh, my wife uses garlic everytime she fixes pasta and linguini. She's half Italian you know, and those Italians can't seem to get enough of their garlic, if you know what I mean."

I explained to him that I was attending the sixty-ninth annual meeting of the National Nutritional Food Association, which was the largest organization of health food retailers and manufacturers in the country. And that it was being held the weekend of July 14–16, 1995, in "the gaming capital of the world." "Health food, yeh," the officer said in an ungrammatical fashion. "My mom is into that sorta stuff. She's always popping vitamin pills. Drives my dad nuts sometimes!"

As Lt. Jones whipped out his fairly well-used-up ticket book, he sort of carelessly waved it in the air, remarking at the same time: "Would you believe that this is my *third* book for the week? Must have written 78 tickets so far on this stretch of road. I like it the best, because this is where I catch most motorists exceeding the limit."

The Cop with the Colitis

"Say, maybe you could help me out with something," he said in earnestness as he began copying information from my driver's license into his book. "I'm bothered with a bowel disease that the doctor calls colitis. Ever hear of it?" I nodded that I did.

"I get these bloody discharges sometimes when I make a trip to the can," he continued. "And get pain in my gut, right about here [motioning with his hand towards his abdomen]. And I've been dropping some in my weight. My vision seems to be okay, but wrist and fingers get a little stiff every now and then."

"*That* last symptom might come from writing so darned many tickets," I added dryly.

"Hey, you're a pretty good, Doc," he laughed. "I like your sense of humor a lot. But is there anything you can tell me that will help me over this?"

"Maybe," I said with some reservation, "provided you help me with *that* problem" (while at the same time pointing with my finger at his ticket book).

Some Remedies for the Big Guy with the Badge

I encouraged him to cease drinking coffee and milk for a while until his condition showed signs of clearing up. "I bet you're a 'meat and potatoes' kind of guy," I speculated. He nodded that he was. I further admonished him to lay off all fried or charbroiled meats for a while. He groaned at this suggestion. But I helped ease his psychological pain a little by adding that he could continue to eat *some* red meat and fish, provided it was baked, steamed, or stewed, "And you must chew every single mouthful very carefully before swallowing," I cautioned. "Half-digested animal protein appears to be part of your overall problem."

By now I had his complete attention, for he had paused in writing up my ticket. "Have you ever heard of papaya juice?" I asked. He nodded in the affirmative. "Then I advise you to buy some bottled quarts of this juice from any Smith's or Albertson's supermarkets. You should also get some ripe bananas or else have your wife do this for you." Next, I asked him if he had a food blender in his home. He responded that they did and thought it was a Vita-Mix whole-food machine, but didn't know for sure.

"My wife just bought one recently," he added, "after getting some literature in the mail regarding it. It's probably the one you mentioned, though."

I instructed him to put one half of a peeled, ripe banana into the Vita-Mix container and then add $1/_2$ cup papaya juice and blend with the lid on for two minutes. "Drink a glass of this with *every* meal you eat," I told him.

And between meals he could drink a nice blend of chamomile and cinnamon tea, which would provide additional healing comfort for his problem. I told him how to bring a pint of water to a boil and then add two cinnamon sticks and reduce the heat to simmer stage for a few minutes. He then was instructed to add $1^1/_2$ tablespoons of chamomile flowers, cover with a lid, remove from the stove, and steep for 30 minutes. The tea was to be strained while still warm. He was to drink one cup of this delicious herb tea twice daily on an empty stomach.

Because he couldn't remember everything I had said, he asked if I would write it down and gave me a piece of paper and pen on which to do so. He thanked me for giving him some good advice that would help him a lot. Then he finished filling out the ticker, tore my copy from his book, and handed it to me without ever asking me to sign it. "I'm going to let you off easy this time and just give you a warning instead," he replied. "But if I were you I'd stay within the speed limit, Doc. It's a lot safer, and you won't be meeting more of my buddies down the line who aren't as kind-hearted as I've been with you."

We shook hands and parted, having assisted each other with our respective problems.

Hiatal Hernia and Heartburn Disappear

Ever had one of those famous "Maalox Moments" as routinely advertised on television? Well, count yourself lucky if you haven't. But for millions of Americans who constantly suffer from hiatal hernia or heartburn, an agent such as Maalox or Tums has proven to be almost indispensable.

Menstrual Cramping Relieved

Renee is an executive secretary with an insurance company. She is 37 years of age, but manifests symptoms frequently associated with premenstrual syndrome. Abdominal cramping is one of the most common of them. She had tried just about everything for it, until we met at a National Health Federation convention held in Pittsburgh in the early part of June 1995.

I was there lecturing, and she was in attendance to listen to a number of her favorite speakers. By accident, she came into the wrong room expecting to hear a holistic gynecologist speak on women's problems and instead ended up staying to hear me speak on the healing benefits of juices.

She was intrigued with my recommended therapy program for menstrual cramping consisting of papaya juice and chamomile tea. She bought some bottled juice and packaged tea from a local health food store. She drank one glass of the fruit juice every day and two cups of the *warm* tea made according to the directions on the package label.

She later wrote to thank me for helping relieve her PMS symptoms, especially the cramping.

Insomnia Taken Care of

Life is full of little ironies. Consider this one, if you will—it's a real hoot, but absolutely true. Jack Worthen is a salesman for a local mattress factory outlet in Salt Lake City. But he constantly complained to his friends and relatives about not being able to get a good night's sleep, even though one would think he could, considering his profession.

But now comes a remedy from nature that is even more effective. And besides relieving the symptoms, it can actually help to heal the problems, too. I'm speaking of bottled papaya juice and how effective it has been in helping to remedy that reverse regurgitation effect so common to hiatal hernia or that bloated gas feeling that's indicative of heartburn.

With every meal, I counsel those who suffer from either of these to drink one-half cup of papaya juice *slowly;* don't gulp it down in a hurry if you want it to do some good. I have never known this remedy to fail to work when properly and consistently used.

Jack was referred to me by a friend of a friend. Before I had a chance to start speaking, the man held up his hand and emphatically stated: "P-l-e-a-s-e don't start off by telling me to get myself a more comfortable mattress. I've not only heard that a thousand times over, but have tried using a number of mattresses without very much success. With that over, you can now speak."

I told Jack about chamomile and how much it had helped people like him who suffered from insomnia. "Some of the chemical constituents in it," I noted, "are like 'herbal lullabies' and help to put the brain to sleep in no time at all." He was quite excited to try it. I added that "chamomile tea only works for this particular problem if it is taken in the form of a *warm tea!*"

About five days later, he called my home early in the morning and exclaimed with obvious joy: "Doc, you'll never know how much that tea has helped me. I'm getting more sleep now than I've had in ages. That chamomile stuff works like a charm!" (I might add here that whenever people refer to me as "Doc" it's more as a nickname because of my Ph.D. in medical anthropology and *not* because I am a physician or someone who is licensed to treat sick people, which I am definitely *not* in the business of doing!)

Cramps and Lower Back Pain Gone in Minutes

A rather obese fellow who works in the newspaper business went to a local chiropractor in the Salt Lake City area for abdominal cramps and lower back ache. Because of his somewhat expansive girth, the skinny, slightly built chiropractor found it next to impossible to work on him. So he referred him to me in the hopes that there might be something in my extensive herbal repertoire that might do the fellow some good.

I told the man to boil a pint of water and then add up to six whole cinnamon sticks, breaking them up if necessary to fit into the pot. Cover with a lid and gently simmer on low heat, I continued, for up to seven minutes. Then set aside and steep for 40 minutes before straining. He was advised to drink one cup of the warm tea four times daily as well as to apply a hot pack (hand towel soaked in some of the heated tea and wrung out) over his belly and lower back several times each day. He reported back a while later that his symptoms had cleared up within two weeks of doing this.

COMMON COLD

Lady Skydiver Relies on Echinacea Tea to Get Well

DESCRIPTION

A common cold most generally is a minor, self-limited viral infection of the mucosa of the upper respiratory tract, especially in the nose. It is manifested by sneezing, nasal obstruction and discharge, and lasts an average of a week.

A medical survey taken some years ago of 871 people with colds revealed the following general symptoms, ranked according to the frequency of their appearance:

nasal inflammation (head cold and sneezing) 50–66%

sore throat, nearly 50%

hoarseness and cough, between 25–50%

headache 25%

muscular aches, lethargy, and malaise varied between 25 and 45%

fever and chills varied anywhere from 15 to 30%

Free-Falling from 3,500 Feet in the Air

Rosie O'Toole is quite a lady! This 38-year-old woman is unflappable even when she's free-falling from a height of 4,000 feet or less *above ground.* How does she manage to stay so calm while jumping out of an airplane in midair, I wondered. "Oh, that's simple," she told me. "I just silently chant my mantra and meditate, pretending that I've been reincarnated into a bird. Then nothing bothers me, even when everything else on the ground looks like flyspecks to me."

Rosie often catches a cold, not from someone else around her but whenever she is way up high doing her stuff. "Maybe I'm susceptible to something up there," she joked with a finger pointed skyward. You see, this woman does skydiving in her spare time and probably doesn't bundle up well enough to withstand the frigid temperatures in the upper atmosphere. "Oh, I dress warmly enough," she admitted, "but probably let my immune system run down more than I should."

Rosie explained to me what entailed a typical skydive. "We go through the usual safety equipment check," she began. "Then we board our aircraft for the flight up. The main chutes we use are always attached to a line in the compartment of our plane that usually takes us up to around 3,500 feet.

"Once we jump out of the door, our main chutes are automatically pulled open. Then we start our lazy drift earthward. Simple movements like pulling down the shrouds (those are the cords that connect my harness to the canopy) right or left give me directional control.

"When hitting the ground a few minutes later, I never land squarely on my feet. Instead, I've learned how to roll *into* the ground, going shoulders first, to prevent impact injury. Then I get up, run to my chute to pound the air out of it, and wait for our transportation to take us back to the airport."

When I asked her what it felt like, she thought for a moment and then replied: "It's the ultimate adrenaline rush! It sure beats the hell out of bungee-cord jumping!"

Rosie's Cure for the Common Cold

"So," I asked her with some obvious mischief in my voice, "what does the 'high-flying Rosie O'Toole' do whenever she feels a cold coming on?" Then, being unable to resist further mirth, I added: "I guess for you that would be considered a 'bad *air* day.'"

She chuckled and said, "Well, John, there's nothing like a warm cup of brew to clear out your head." More specifically, she meant the herbal blend from Traditional Medicinals called Echinacea Plus. "This stuff has both kinds of echinacea in it," she said reading from the package label, "plus lemongrass and spearmint. I take about five *hot* cups of it, one every three hours, whenever I'm feeling crappy. It usually doesn't take too long—maybe 24 or 36 hours if I can get lots of rest—before I'm back on my feet again, wanting to free-fall."

GET WELL TONIC

> *8 teabags Echinacea Plus (available at most health food stores or herb shops)*
>
> *1¹/₂ pints spring or mineral water*
>
> *2 tbsp. fresh-squeezed lemon juice*
>
> *1 tsp. chopped licorice root bark*
>
> *1 tsp. pure vanilla flavoring*

Boil the water. Add the licorice root bark, cover, and simmer on low heat for 3 minutes. Pour (but do not strain) into a teapot. Add the teabags. Cover and steep 20 minutes. Strain and reheat tea. Add lemon juice and vanilla flavoring. Drink very warm.

Rosie also believes in taking some vitamin A (50,000 I.U.), vitamin C (3,500 mg.), and Kyolic Garlic (3 capsules) *twice* daily on an empty stomach. And if her throat feels a little sore, she uses some bee propolis from Montana Naturals. "I just tilt my head back as far as I can," she said, showing me how it was done, "and squirt some of this stuff in the very back of my throat. It burns a little, but otherwise won't hurt you. I don't advise getting it on the tongue 'cause of the awful taste, though."

If your local health food store doesn't have the Echinacea Plus tea blend or another equally good product, Cold Care P.M., call Traditional Medicinals in Sebastopol, California, at (707) 823-8911. Likewise, if you can't find the bee propolis mentioned here, call Montana Naturals in Arlee, Montana, at (406) 726-3214 to get it.

CONSTIPATION

The Old Standby Still Works—Prune Juice

DESCRIPTION

I composed the following ditty especially for the readers of this book. It pretty much reflects just how actively prunes can work in the gut in a matter of minutes. It also livens these pages up with a little bit of humor.

ODE TO PRUNES

Prunes, prunes, the magic fruit,
The more you eat, the more you toot.
And the more you toot, the better you'll feel,
So you oughta have prunes for every meal!

Prune juice, prune juice, works quite well
When your colon starts to smell,
Swig it down without any fear,
And have that blockage disappear!

So, now that you've tried it
Stay close to a toilet,
'Cuz those prunes will keep on working still
Or else you'll end up with a cleaning bill!

© 1995 John Heinerman

"Old Reliable" Never Fails

I've been the editor of *Utah Prime Times,* the Beehive State's largest seniors newspaper, for six years as of 1996. Since our main readership is those people who are age 50 and older, I'm always on the prowl for human-interest stories that involve older folks. A part of my spare time is spent visiting seniors centers and rest homes throughout the state looking for things to write about.

In the Rocking Chair Rest Haven, located in one Utah city, I met a spunky lady nicknamed Big Bertha. "I'm like one of those big guns on them battle ships the Navy uses in wartime," she said. "I'm packing lots of power behind my size." This 65-year-old woman stands 5-foot-9-inches tall and weighs in at 237 pounds. "I'm *all* woman!" she brags in a naughty sort of way.

We got to talking about this and that and the other. Eventually, our long-winded conversation drifted into the purpose of my visit there, namely home remedies. "Yes," she exclaimed matter-of-factly, "I got something for your paper." In our newspaper we have a special section that I introduced several years ago devoted to health topics; it is called the "Mature Health" section. What she intended to tell me would sooner or later show up in this part of the newspaper.

She proceeded to tell me how badly she used to suffer from constipation and how she tried virtually every laxative under the sun. "If it was meant to move bowels, then rest assured, *Sonny,* I probably tried it," she said gleefully. Finding nothing worked to her satisfaction, she decided to drink some prune juice.

"When they [meaning the staff at the rest home] take some of us out to go shopping once a week," she continued, "I bought me some of this juice at the local supermarket. I got the kind that *includes* some of the pulp. I figured it would help me better." She started drinking *two* full 8-ounce glasses of this morning and evening. Within days her constipation was gone and, according to her now, "I've been regular ever since. Works like a charm, it does."

COUGHING

When You Bark Like a Dog, Take Dogwood

DESCRIPTION

There are a number of reliable herbs that have been used for count-less years by many herbalists for the treatment of coughs. Among them are included such well-known remedies as horehound, lemon, lobelia, onion, radish, slippery elm, yarrow, white pine, and wild cherry. Lesser known plants for allaying coughing spells have includ-ed asafoetida and marijuana, of all things.

Not too long ago, I learned about another remedy that isn't as well known as some of these others might be. But, boy, is it ever effec-tive. I'm speaking of the flowering dogwood tree, which is found from Maine to Florida and west to Minnesota, Kansas, and Texas. The bark is rough and brown and has been used in times past as a suitable substitute for quinine.

Correctly Identifying Your Cough

There are two basic types of cough: one that is dry and another that is wet. A dry cough usually is nonproductive, while a wet one will produce considerable matter. In other words, a dry cough is a hack-ing sound without anything coming up, whereas a wet cough will yield sputum. Knowing *which* kind you have enables you to know how much flowering dogwood bark tea to take.

Leonard's Cough Remedy

Leonard Mays lives in southeastern Kentucky. He considers himself "a ge-noo-wine hill-billy." I met him a while back during a routine investigation of residents in his "holler"—that's that slang term for the kind of hollow located between two hills that many people in Kentucky live in. Leonard's folks have been using flowering dogwood, he told me, "ever since the cows cum home by themselves."

He claimed a tea made from the bark was good for coughs often associated with colds, croup, emphysema, laryngitis, pleurisy, fever, tuberculosis (TB), bronchitis, asthma, the flu, pneumonia, and, of course, real whooping cough. "My pappy used to take it all the time himself, when he would cough his head off like a damn fool," Leonard stated. "And Ma, why she used to give it to us young-uns if we started soundin' like our hunting dogs." He noted that it usually took no more than two cups "to git us to quite down agin."

LEONARD'S "MOONSHINE" TEA

You're probably wondering why I'm calling this "moonshine" tea. It seems that's how my informant always fixes it—"the best tea *always* has a little moonshine in it," he bragged.

> **one pint water**
>
> **1–2 tbsp. dried flowering dogwood bark**
>
> **1 tsp. sourmash whiskey or bourbon per cup**

Boil the water. Add the bark. Cover and simmer on low heat for 10 minutes. Set aside and steep for 40 minutes. Strain only one cup at a time. Reheat until rather warm, but not too hot. Add the liquor to the cup, stir, and slowly drink. Tilt the head back and gargle the throat with a little of it, before swallowing. Always drink it on an empty stomach.

CRAMPS

The Pause that Refreshes—Iced Tea

DESCRIPTION

The way things are currently going, it probably won't be too long before busboys in Boston, New York, and San Francisco patrol restaurants pouring iced tea instead of the customary water. This is currently the trend in Atlanta, New Orleans, and Charleston, and seems to be spreading. Julian Niccolini, the manager of the Four Seasons in Manhattan, told me a while back, "It looks as if more of our customers are drinking iced tea than anything else with their lunches these days. Must be some kinda trend, I guess."

This particularly southern thirst-quencher is becoming an annual phenomenon across the country. On any given day during the spring, summer, and fall months, almost 129 million Americans will be drinking tea; about 20 percent fewer than this continue to drink it even in the cooler months of the year. These statistics are based on research done by the Tea Council, a trade group. And they say that the iced variety accounts for nearly 80 percent of all the tea consumed in this country, up from 70 percent in 1980. In 1960, less that 50 percent of the tea consumed was iced. The Tea Council is looking to make some serious inroads into the gigantic soft-drink market, where Americans easily consume more than 45 gallons of the stuff per capita.

Healthier for You?

The boom in ready-to-drink iced tea seems to be part of the fitness craze these days. In the huge beverage industry, iced tea is commonly called an "alternative beverage"—lighter, more refreshing, and more natural than cloying carbonated soft drinks loaded with sugar or artificial sweeteners and preservatives.

There seems to be a general perspective among the public that iced tea is a suitable alternative to soft drinks. Younger, more health-conscious Americans are being drawn to it. Iced teas fill a growing demand for a noncarbonated beverage that, unlike water, has some flavor but is not as "heavy" as fruit juice.

But in spite of their appeal to the fitness crowd, some segments of our society might not appreciate what else is in iced teas. Twelve ounces of iced tea has 22 to 26 milligrams of caffeine, compared with

36 to 45 milligrams for cola drinks and 90 to 200 milligrams for coffee. For coffee drinkers and cola guzzlers, this might come as welcome news, but certainly not to devout Mormons or Seventh-Day Adventists. In fact, both religious groups have very strict codes of health that strongly prohibit the consumption of caffeinated beverages in *any* form.

Teas for Two

There are several iced teas I'd like to recommend that have proven quite useful in remedying abdominal cramps or leg cramps (sometimes called "Charley horses") and muscles spasms. I like to think of them as "teas for two." They are ready-to-drink Nestea, Lipton Original Iced Tea, and Lipton Brisk Iced Tea. Between one and two cups sipped *slowly* through a plastic straw will usually allay the worst cramps or spasms within about 20 minutes.

Home Brew Your Own Iced Teas

Strong black teas, delicate varieties, herbal teas, and flavored teas all make wonderfully delicious iced teas. The best sweeteners for them are either pure maple syrup, pure vanilla flavor, clover honey, or brown sugar. Fruit juice or ice cubes made of juice are nice additions, as are lemon wedges, crushed berries, or sprigs of mint.

In areas of the country where the water may be tainted with too much chloride or fluoride, I suggest you use spring or mineral water out of a bottle. There are two methods for making iced tea: traditional and cold-water.

The Traditional Way. Bring one quart of cold water to a rolling boil in a nonreactive saucepan. Remove it from the heat and add 6 teaspoons of loose tea or 6 tea bags of your favorite blend. Cover the pot and steep 7 minutes. Then strain the brewed tea into a pitcher and add two cups of cold water. Pour over ice into a tall glass and enjoy.

The Cold-Water Method. Put 6 teaspoons of loose tea or 6 tea bags in a pitcher and add 6 cups of cool water. Cover loosely, set aside for $4^{1}/_{2}$ hours, then refrigerate. Strain the tea and serve it over ice, or refrigerate again.

Don't make herbal tea this way. Instead, steep it in boiling water for about 15 minutes.

Some think that the cold-water method prevents iced tea from becoming cloudy. While not detracting from the flavor of the tea, the muddy look that a glass pitcher of refrigerated iced tea acquires doesn't enhance its eye appeal by any means.

CROHN'S DISEASE

Mother Makes Terrific Recovery with Aloe/ Carrot Juice Combo

DESCRIPTION

Aloe vera has been extensively studied by scientists worldwide for its wonderful healing properties. Aloe vera is an especially effective, safe, and cheap remedy for burns, wounds, and internal inflammations. The mucilaginous gel in the parenchymatous tissue of plant leaf centers is responsible for this healing action. The gel is 96 percent water and contains numerous polysaccharides. One of them is a glucomannan quite similar in composition to another polysaccharide found in guar and locust bean gums.

Besides polysaccharides, the remaining 4 percent of the gel is composed of organic acids, amino acids, antibiotic principles, and "biogenic stimulators." There are also trace amounts of certain minerals, such as zinc and selenium, saponins or soapy compounds, steroids, and enzymes. I strongly believe that it is chemical interactions between these four constituents (minerals, saponins, steroids, and enzymes) that give the aloe gel its marvelous healing properties.

The gel is prepared in different ways, one of them being in liquid form, so it can be taken internally.

Carrots are very rich in beta-carotene (a form of vitamin A) and natural sugars. When used in conjunction with aloe vera liquid, carrots can help reduce intestinal inflammation.

Remarkable Recovery from Intestinal Inflammation

Gina Mitchell, aged 23, is a young mother residing with her husband in Pleasant Grove, Utah (about 25 miles south of Salt Lake City). They have two young children, 3 years and 1 year old. But in spite of a happy marriage and two wonderful kids, Gina has been in a lot of pain.

Until recently, Gina suffered from Crohn's disease, which is an idiopathic inflammatory disorder of the small intestine and colon involving layers of the bowel. It began as a slow, progressive disease with her, causing obstruction of the bowel, fistulization, and inflammation of adjacent structures. Other sites within her gastrointestinal tract were also affected by it.

This idiopathic inflammation can occur in all forms of Crohn's, or as small-bowel disease or colon disease only, or a combination of colon and small-bowel disease. Gina's symptoms included periodic diarrhea, some abdominal pain, minor weight loss, limited spondylitis (vertebrae inflammation) and arthritis, a little iritis (iris inflammation), and occasional abdominal mass.

Her doctor prescribed Prednisone 20 to 40 mg. daily for the first 3 weeks with a tapering after that in the fourth to sixth weeks of treatment. But this drug produced an untoward side effect in that her face swelled dramatically and became somewhat moon-shaped.

Gina's mom, Irene Remund, first told me of her daughter's condition and had me contact the man who helped Gina get well again.

On Saturday, July 22, 1995, I spoke by phone with Ron Stokes of Pleasant Grove, Utah. "I'm not really an herbalist or nutritionist," he freely admitted. "I'm just a retired federal government employee who worked as an engineer for ten years in the Department of Labor. I'll be 70 very soon and got my present knowledge from reading self-improvement health books, such as the kind you write, Dr. Heinerman." But he couldn't recall necessarily reading any of mine.

"When her mom first told me about Gina's condition, I encouraged the young lady to try aloe vera juice. But like so many young people who aren't too well acquainted with natural remedies, she just turned up her nose at the suggestion. That is, until her symptoms started getting worse. Then she began to listen more earnestly to what I had to say. Funny, isn't it, how it sometimes takes a little pain and suffering to get someone to listen to good advice?" Ron thoughtfully mused.

Ron recommended that she buy a gallon of *liquid* aloe vera in the quart size. Gina took about $1/4$ cup of this with every meal, morning, noon, and night, for three weeks. Her facial swelling and diarrhea started to go away. She then decided, on her own, to add the liquid aloe vera to a special "vegetable cocktail" she devised. In one of those juicing machines from the Stone Age, she juiced 10 carrots, 6 stalks of celery, 1 green bell pepper, and 2 small apples. The down side to using a cumbersome juicer like this is that it discards the valuable pulp, not to mention that it takes a lot of time to clean and reassemble.

Twice a day, Gina would drink a 6-fluid-ounce glass of this "vegetable cocktail" with $1/4$ cup of liquid aloe vera stirred in. Her pain and intestinal discomforts had nearly all cleared up within a period of two months from the time she began this simple back-to-nature program of healing. Her doctor was wonderfully amazed at her recovery and attributed it to the Prednisone, while she knew better, but kept this little "health secret" to herself.

Energy When You Need It

Ron told me that he likes to ride trail bikes cross country "in the roughest terrain we can find." During the middle of August 1995, a group of seniors he belongs to decided to retrace the original Pony Express trail across Utah and Nevada. They started out at the State Line Casino in Wendover, Utah, and eventually ended up in western Nevada somewhere.

Ron said that to prepare himself for this long and arduous trip, "I'm starting to drink a mixed greens-carrot-juice combo myself. I find it gives me the energy and vitality I need for an adventure such as this."

Prevents Bone and Muscle Injuries

Furthermore, Ron confirmed, "This type of activity is really quite punishing on the body. It's so physically demanding that unless you're in really good shape, you can end up with bruised muscles (especially in the buttocks) and strained ligaments and tendons (in the calves and ankles). Most of these likely injuries would result from the jarring ride of the trail bike itself. We're not talking a nice, big, comfortable Harley Davidson here, by any means; we're talking rough riding on a trail bike, for sure. And sometimes, when these bikes slide out from under you on sand or gravel, the rider can sustain a bone fracture.

"So, by taking plenty of this mixed greens-carrot juice combination well in advance of our trip," he added, "I'm only toughening up my body muscles and bones and reducing my risk of sustained injury." His final comment was given with a good-natured laugh: "When you're no longer a 'spring chicken' but more like an 'old rooster,' then you gotta take something that will help you stay in shape. And these juices are my ticket to good health!"

Promotes Bowel Elimination More Easily

One final comment to everything Mr. Stokes said. It has been my experience through the years in drinking carrot juice every so often that it wonderfully promotes bowel movements, no matter how constipated you may be. I usually drink about a quart of the stuff when I'm driving long distances and can testify that within a few hours I can expect to answer "nature's call."

CRYING (UNCONTROLLABLE)

How One Woman Conquered Her Moods of Weeping

DESCRIPTION

Most of the self-care health books on the market today do not give any specific information with regard to the emotion of crying. Either the authors don't think it's important enough to mention in their works or else they fail to connect it with any kind of serious disorder. In a survey my staff and I did of 57 such books at the Anthropological Research Center in Salt Lake City some time ago, we found only two of them with scant information on this topic.

The type of crying dealt with here isn't the kind that is normally associated with joy or grief. Rather it is the emotional response that is common to manic depression (now called bipolar disorder). According to the *Comprehensive Textbook of Psychiatry* (5th Edition) edited by Harold I. Kaplan, M.D., and Benjamin J. Sadock, M.D. (Baltimore: Williams and Wilkin, 1989), uncontrollable crying is frequent in cases of bipolar disorder type II. Females are two to three times more likely to have such mood disorders as males are.

Herbs Helped Her Resume a Normal Life Again

Patricia Hupp of Atlanta, Georgia, is a medical technician. She is 34 years of age, twice divorced, with two children (a boy 15 and a girl 16). She was diagnosed some years ago as having bipolar disorder II. She would be very productive at work for a week or longer, then suddenly and unexpectedly bottom out with another bout of severe depression.

Patricia characterized her hypomania this way: "I could go for days without much sleep and accomplish an incredible amount of work, much to my own amazement. Then, without warning, I'd sink into this deep emotional pit. Not only would I feel like sleeping all day long, but I would sometimes start crying for no apparent reason. It was very embarrassing, to say the least. My doctor had me on lithium citrate." (This was formerly used in soft drinks, by the way.)

She admitted that while the medication did help to some extent, her sleeping remained erratic, and periodic outbursts of weeping were still a common thing. So, Patricia started reading up on herbs and decided to try two in particular, stinging nettle and chamomile. She took them as warm teas every day for an entire month. During this time she noticed that her sleeping dramatically improved. More important, though, "my crying stopped just as suddenly as it had begun." This especially pleased her very much.

"The reason I'm letting you use my name and giving you this information for your book," she told me, "is because I want other women out there who may be suffering from the same things to know that there really is *something* they can do about bipolar disorder besides conventional drug therapy."

WEEP-No-More Teas

1 pint boiling water

2 tbsp. stinging nettle or chamomile

Add either herb, cover, set aside, and steep 20 minutes. Drink one cup of *warm* tea twice daily. Do this with *both* teas. Make separate batches of each tea every day. Alternate the intake throughout the day.

CYSTITIS

(see Bladder Infection)

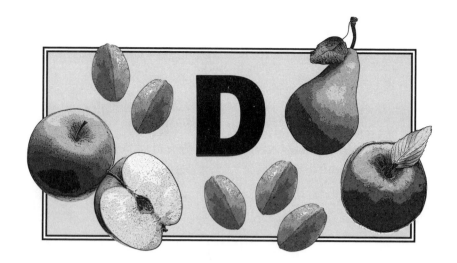

DEPRESSION

(see Anxiety, Insomnia, and Mood Swings)

DIABETES

A Tonic Duo for Hyperglycemia

DESCRIPTION

Diabetes comes in two varieties: diabetes insipidus and diabetes mellitus. The first is marked by large amounts of urine production in the body regardless of how much fluid is consumed. The other kind results from the production of insufficient amounts of insulin by the pancreas. This diabetes is divided into two categories. Type I is known either as insulin-dependent diabetes mellitus or as juvenile diabetes; Type II is recognized either as noninsulin-dependent diabetes or as adult-onset diabetes.

Life-Saving Teas

In my nearly quarter century of research on empirical folk medicine, I've discovered that two common herbs work best for treating diabetes. They are alfalfa leaves and fenugreek seed, and they should be used as teas. They help the pancreas to produce more insulin. An average of two cups per day of *each* tea is recommended. Alternate their intake with meals.

ALFALFA TEA

1 pint water (distilled or spring)
2 tbsp. dried alfalfa leaves

Boil the water. Add the leaves. Stir and cover. Set aside and steep 20 minutes. Strain and drink.

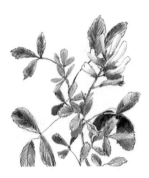

FENUGREEK TEA

1 pint water (distilled or spring)
2 tsp. seeds

Boil the water. Add the seeds. Cover and simmer on low heat for 4 minutes. Set aside and steep 15 minutes. Strain and drink.

DERMATITIS

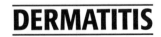

(see Eczema)

DIARRHEA

World War II G.I. Remedy Used by the "King of the Blues"

DESCRIPTION

Corn has always been thought of primarily as being a food of all Native Americans in this hemisphere. While this is correct, it is also true that corn has been a regular staple of many African-Americans and their early slave ancestors. In his curious little work, *Ethno-Botany of the Black Americans* (Algonac, MI: Reference Publications, Inc., 1979, pp. 196–199) author William Grimé explained how slaves living on Virginia plantations a couple of centuries ago made a type of hasty pudding from corn, which "the Negroes [eat] with cider, hog's lard, or molasses. Furthermore, ". . . in the southern states . . . each Negro is allowed a peck [of corn] in a week for his sustenance."

A Remedy from B. B. King

Just about all people know who B. B. King is. If they don't, then they've probably been out of touch with the human race for a while now. In 1995 King celebrated his seventieth birthday, on September 16. He was introduced into the Blues Foundation Hall of Fame in 1984 and the Rock 'n' Roll Hall of Fame in 1988. He became an influential, five time Grammy-winning star with more than 126 albums to his credit. In addition to all this, he has received four honorary doctorates and was a founding member of the John F. Kennedy Performing Arts Center.

King is to blues what Einstein was to relativity—the man and his music are virtually inseparable. (Blues is a particular style of music originating with southern Blacks, expressing melancholy and exhibiting a repetition of blue notes in both melody and harmony.) King was in Salt Lake City performing at Abravanel Hall on Sunday, October 29, 1995, when I caught up with him for a few minutes of interview in my capacity as editor of *Utah Prime Times* (the state's largest monthly seniors' newspaper).

An aunt of his introduced King to guitars, and an uncle who was a man of the cloth taught him basic chords. Still another aunt let the boy listen to Blind Lemon Jefferson and Lonnie Johnson records;

141

they made lasting influences on his life. When he turned 15, B. B. bought his own guitar for $8 and quickly mastered the instrument before forming his own group, a gospel quartet.

But it was during World War II that King, while serving a stint in the Army in an all-black company, was first introduced to jazz and blues. By the time he was discharged in the mid-'40s, he had a large repertoire.

The man wanted to talk blues, but I wanted to talk a little bit about folk remedies. So I interrupted him to ask if he knew of any folk remedies that might have worked for him or for his family in his lifetime.

He recalled that while he was in the Army there was an old cook working in the mess-hall kitchen who had come up with a pretty good remedy for diarrhea, which a lot of the guys in the unit seemed to suffer from. The joke, of course, that circulated among the enlisted men was that their diarrhea came from this cook's food, and because of the many complaints getting back to him, he invented a cure for it.

The cook took an unspecified amount of black coffee and so many ears of corn and boiled them all together in a big pot for a couple of hours until they were "done up right" (whatever that means). Then the old cook would strain the liquid out and bottle it in gallon glass jugs and refrigerate it. Whenever any of the G.I.s complained of diarrhea he would have the men drink a couple cups of this brew.

"It was pretty potent stuff as I recall," B. B. remembered. "A man could stomach only a little of it at a time. But it seemed to do the job for everyone concerned."

Then he got back to talking about his music again. "I heard an electric guitar that wasn't playing spiritual," he continued. "It was T-Bone Walker doing 'Stormy Monday,' and that was the prettiest sound I think I ever heard in my life. That's what really started me to play the blues." The blues gave King a ticket out of the drudgery of farm work. And in 1947 he hitchhiked to Memphis to live with a cousin, blues artist Bukka White.

As a free-lance performer, King sang commercials on black radio station WDID and found work under the name Riley King, the "Blues Boy from Beale Street." He soon shortened that to Blues Boy King and finally to the present moniker of B. B.

His first recording in 1949, "Three O'Clock Blues," made the national R&B lists in 1950. By the later 1970s, King was an established star, helped in part by British rockers who had fallen in love with him and the blues. He opened that decade with a gold single, "The Thrill Is Gone."

I changed the subject back again to remedies long enough to ask him if there were anything else he could tell me about folk medicine in his family. He shook his head, mentioning only about the Army remedy and reminding me that it worked best when the soldiers drank the liquid *cold,* never warm. Then, in mock exasperation he asked me, "Kin we git back to talkin' 'bout music again?"

King felt that every professional should be respected for his or her own particular talents. "Blues is what I do best," he stated very matter-of-factly. "Mozart and Beethoven are best known for their classical stuff, [Frank] Sinatra for his, and so forth. So, why can't I have that kind of recognition in what I'm good at, in the blues?"

I told him that his style of music wasn't for me, though it may be for many other people. He laughed hard, looked me straight in the eye, and said, "Son, it doesn't matter if you're black, white, brown, yellow, red, blue, rich, or poor—we *all* have some of the blues in us."

DIARRHEA DRINK FOR G.I. JOES

I experimented around a little with the ingredients King had given me until I came up with this home version of the Army cook's anti-diarrhea tonic.

> *1 quart water*
>
> *1¹/₂ cups coffee grounds (regular, not decaf)*
>
> *1 ear of corn cut into several small sections*

Bring the water to a rolling boil. Add the coffee first; cover and simmer on low heat for about 30 minutes. Lift off the lid and add the corn. Cover again and simmer for another half hour. Then set aside to cool for 30 minutes. Strain and refrigerate. Drink 2 cups every few hours on an empty stomach until the problem clears up.

DIGESTIVE DISTURBANCES

(see Heartburn, Indigestion, Peptic Ulcer)

DIVERTICULITIS

Alleviating the Distress with Czech Remedy

DESCRIPTION

Diverticulosis is a medical condition characterized by the formation of diverticula—small pouchlike herniations along the wall of the G.I. tract. Ordinarily, diverticula appear in the colon, but they have been known to get as far up as the throat in rare instances, believe it or not. It is estimated by some doctors who keep track of disease statistics that *half* of all Americans over the age of 50 have diverticulosis, even though many may not be aware of it.

Czech the Problem this Way

Some years ago a doctor by the name of Jaroslav Kresánek in Bratislava, in what was then the old Czechoslovakia (now two separate countries), used several different herbal tea tonics to correct the symptoms of bloating, gas, nausea, constipation, diarrhea, and lower left abdominal pain or tenderness that are usually associated with diverticulitis.

He made a tea consisting of the roots of licorice and marshmallow and plantain leaf, which he gave to his patients several times throughout the day. In every instance, their symptoms went away and they felt a lot better thereafter.

CZECH TONIC FOR INFLAMMATION

1 1/2 quarts spring or distilled water

1 tbsp. EACH licorice root, marshmallow root, and plantain leaves

1/4 tsp. pure maple syrup (per cup serving)

Boil the water; add the roots, cover and simmer for 10 minutes. Then add the leaves. Stir, cover, and set aside to steep for 40 minutes. Strain. Take 3/4 cup 5 times daily, if necessary, on an empty stomach.

DYSENTERY

Two Herbal Tea Remedies from
Early Mormon Pioneers

DESCRIPTION

Dysentery can be any of a variety of disorders characterized by intestinal inflammation, especially of the colon. It is always attended by severe abdominal pain, straining during bowel movement efforts, and frequent stools containing blood and mucus. The condition can be induced by irritants, bacteria, protozoa, or parasitic worms due to bad water or contaminated food.

The early Latter-Day Saints, like so many other American pioneers of their time, migrated westward into unfamiliar country where good water and food weren't always available. More often than not they would have to make do with whatever water or food was on hand or was found along the way. In many cases the water especially wasn't fit for human consumption, but they had to drink it or die of thirst. For these reasons many of them frequently suffered from dysentery.

Famous Mormon Poetess Cured with Cranesbill

Cranesbill (also called wild geranium or alum root) is a North American wood plant with rose-purple flowers and seeds bearing large, clawlike hooks. It was a common herbal remedy employed by medicine men among the Iroquois for treating cold sores of the lips or mouth, mitigating fevers, healing tomahawk and arrow wounds suffered in battles, and for relief of general malaise. The roots are a very rich source of tannic acid, a potent astringent.

During the early winter and spring of 1846, the majority of Latter-Day Saints began making the slow, long, arduous trek from their warm and cozy homes in Nauvoo, Illinois, to the very uninviting and forlorn Iowa wilderness that lay before them. At a temporary makeshift settlement named Mount Pisgah, Eliza R. Snow became very sick with what one woman historian has characterized as "a form of dysentery."

Because of the wet weather, damp climate, brackish water, and scarcity of food, Eliza accurately characterized the whole situation in

145

these blunt terms: "It is a growling, grumbling, devilish, sickly time with us now." To combat her diarrhea suffered from the dysentery, she resorted to using an old Indian remedy that had proven to be a reputable standby for many early western pioneers. In her diary entry of Wednesday, May 13, 1846, she wrote: "My health much improv'd—I think by using a tea made by Cranesbill for a few days past."

Although no other specific details were provided by Ms. Snow as to how she made the tea, other pioneer references of approximately the same period enable us to learn the manner in which such herbal brews were routinely prepared. One pioneer by the name of Zeb Johnson, who was on his way to the gold fields of California with his brother to seek their fortunes, described very briefly in his own diary how he made some unidentified root tea with which to help cure "mountain fever." He wrote as follows under the entry for 28 August, 1850: "Dug some root today—brushed against my pants to git rid of dirt—chopped palmfull an throo it into coffeepot $^1/_2$ full water—let boyle over fire some—drank me 2 cups of this awful tastin' stuff, bitter as gall—but fever broke by nightfall . . . ."

One would assume this was how Ms. Snow might have made her own root tea. Cranesbill or wild geranium root can be up to six inches in length and bearing numerous knobs out of which smaller rootlets grow. Eliza must have gathered it in the springtime when the tannin content is always the highest. To her the fresh root would have been light brown externally and light-colored and somewhat fleshy on the inside. The rootstock should first of all be washed under running water to remove any debris. Then enough is chopped with a heavy, sharp knife on a cutting board to equal $^2/_3$ to $^3/_4$ cup (the equivalent of a handful, I'd say). This is then put into about one pint of boiling water (roughly the equivalent of one-half coffee pot full) and permitted to cook for about 20 minutes to make a really strong tea (about 10 minutes less for a weaker solution). The liquid is then strained and consumed *lukewarm*.

Brigham Tea Saves Men from Certain Death

The second account concerns two men whose lives were undoubtedly saved with the use of Brigham tea during severe bouts of dysentery and diarrhea. It comes from a book entitled *Autobiography of Charles Walter Cottam: "Lest I Forget to Remember"* (Provo, UT: J. Grant Stevenson, 1968, pp. 112–114). Brigham or Mormon tea is a broomlike shrub closely resembling shave grass. It is found in the arid parts of the United States, especially favoring the deserts of the American west and southwest. Countless settlers through the years have picked the jointed, grooved green stems and branches of this shrub in large gunny-sack quantities to take home with them and make into a delicious brew known as Brigham tea (so named after the early Mormon leader Brigham Young, who was said to favor this drink himself).

Charles Cottam's account begins this way:

> Some time later, we were living in New Harmony, Utah. I went to the ranch and back every few days. I took a trail that was quite steep in places but one that I could negotiate on horseback. One very hot day in July I had my wife prepare a lunch. She made sandwiches with pork products—head cheese and scrapple. I tied the lunch on the back of the saddle. The day was very hot and the horse sweat a great deal. Late that afternoon I ate some of my lunch. That night a severe sharp pain struck me as I attempted to lie down in bed. Then I began to purge and soon began to weaken. I kept purging until I thought I couldn't survive the night. I thought that my body would not be found for days and thought about the children who might soon be fatherless.

> Suddenly I thought about Brigham tea and the way it helped me before. A bush of Brigham tea was just in front of me. I made a fire and some live coals were still in the stove. I grabbed some trash and threw it in the stove to make a quick flame. Then I put a handful of Brigham tea and a little water in the frying pan. A few minutes later the tea was poured into a cup. As soon as it was cooled enough that I could drink it, I drank the whole cup of the tea. Pain and purging both stopped immediately. Since then I have used the tea many times effectively. I have recommended it to others who had similar results.

> One case in particular occurred when I was teaching school in Bunkerville, Nevada. A chiropractor moved to that town and we became very well acquainted. He visited our home occasionally, and one time during a visit, I told him of my experience with Brigham tea. A few weeks after that he hurried over to my place. He reminded me that I had told him about an herb that was effective in stopping dysentery. He said, "Tell me where I can get some. This is an emergency. As there was no medical doctor here, a man came to me for help. He has the worst case of dysentery that I have ever known. I have done everything I can for him and he is no better. He will have to be helped soon or he will die."

> I said, "I have some mountain rush [another name for Brigham tea or *Ephedra nevadensis*] here; I keep it on hand all the time." I gave him some and told him how to prepare it. He hurried away and I didn't see him again for a few days. When I did see him, I said, "How is your patient doing?" He replied, "I don't know. I made the tea for him and gave him a drink of it. It stopped his trouble. In a little while later he told me that he felt so much better that he would resume his journey."

These are but a few of the many cases in which I have known mountain rush to be effective in curing summer complaint, diarrhea, and dysentery. There are some who use it in their daily diet for other less drastic troubles.

Note: Readers should not confuse this species of ephedra with that of another type, called mahuang. This Chinese herb contains a potent druglike substance called ephedrine, which has been misused in a number of herbal "uppers" intended to promote euphoria and short bursts of adrenaline strength. But products such as Herbal Ecstasy, which contain this kind of ephedra as well as kola nut, are now being investigated by the Food and Drug Administration and could soon become severely regulated or removed from the market altogether. Brigham tea, though, does *not* contain any ephedrine, and, therefore, is quite safe to use for long periods of time.

BRIGHAM TEA

1 quart spring or distilled water

4 cups Brigham or Mormon tea

some dairy cream or canned milk

honey, molasses, or pure maple syrup to sweeten

Boil the water first. Then add the coarsely cut Brigham tea stems. Cover with lid and simmer on low heat for 10 minutes. Set aside and steep another 20 minutes. Strain and refrigerate. Reheat only the amount desired. Add a little honey or molasses or maple syrup to sweeten while still relatively hot and stir until well blended. Cream or canned milk is optional, but does improve the flavor of the tea. Drink warm with a meal or on an empty stomach. *This is one of the MOST DELICIOUS herbal brews I know.* By my way of thinking, it ranks nearly equal to warm chamomile tea for imaginative and real physical goodness.

DYSFUNCTIONAL UTERINE BLEEDING

Chinese Herbal Tonics Are a Woman's Friend

DESCRIPTION

Dysfunctional uterine bleeding is a condition in which a woman may skip her period often, or may experience frequent bleeding between periods. Doctors are inclined to think that such abnormal patterns are related, a complex interaction between the brain's hypothalamus gland, the ovaries, and the uterus. Anxiety and depression are known to change neurotransmitter levels in the brain, causing a disruption in normal hypothalmic activity patterns. This, in turn, upsets the normal function of a woman's reproductive organs.

Chinese Herbs Took the DYS out of DYS-functional

The following is a true story, but my female informant asked that I not use her name, nor identify the city she lives in. However, she did permit her age and occupation to be mentioned. I have assigned her the pseudonym Gloria X.

Gloria X is a 39-year-old CEO (chief executive officer) of a mid-sized manufacturing company. She told me she spends an average of 65 hours per week in her office or in the board room. "I am a woman on the move, but know where I'm going," she said with apparent self-confidence.

Not too long ago one of her toughest rivals attempted a takeover of her firm through a massive buy-up of the company's stock. Gloria had to look for a "friendly suitor" in the form of another company to help her financially thwart this aggressive takeover. "It was long and hard and difficult," she recalled. "We finally managed to buy back enough of our own stock to give us controlling interest. This discouraged our rivals, and they quietly went away after that. But it sure as hell left me drained and an emotional and physical wreck."

Her first symptoms of dysfunctional uterine bleeding were pretty obvious. Gloria had heavy bleeding for two and a half weeks, followed immediately by *nothing* for seven weeks, and then three days of spotting. "That's pretty much how it went for over two and a half months," she reminded me. "I internalized a lot of anxiety and felt as if I were in an abyss of deep despair."

She came to me because of my reputation in folk medicine. "If anyone can help me, you can," she remarked. She quickly admitted, though, that she knew I was *not* a medical doctor and *not* licensed to prescribe or diagnose. "I know that all you can give me," she continued, "is knowledge belonging to others whom you've interviewed around the world. Now that we've cleared up those formalities," she insisted, "can we get on with the herbs you have in mind for me to use?"

There were several teas I had in mind for her to use. The first was green tea, with which she was familiar. I told her to drink two *warm* cups of it every day, and it would help reduce her anxiety and high blood pressure somewhat. Next I recommended dong quai (also spelled tang kuei) for its energy-boosting properties; I asked her to drink one cup of this each day with her noon meal.

Finally, to stop the incessant bleeding, I advised her to make a tea combination from a plant called pseudoginseng (San Qí in the Mandarin dialect) and the pollen scraped from cattails or pussywillows (Pu Húang). A couple of the items she had to get through an Oriental food market and Chinese herb shop.

She made them the way I instructed and faithfully took them all for six weeks. After being on these tonics for only a couple of weeks, she called to congratulate me on "a job well done" and said, "You sure know your stuff when it comes to herbs." Her periods were already starting to get back to normal again, but she intended to take these teas a little longer just to be on the safe side.

Tonics for the Uterus

Readers are encouraged to check the last part of the entry on CAVITIES for directions to making green tea.

To Make Dong Quai Tea: Boil 1 pint of spring or distilled water. Add 2 teaspoons of angelica or dong quai root. Cover with a lid, simmer 3 minutes, then set aside and steep for 12 minutes. Strain and drink one cup twice daily: once before breakfast and again before dinner.

To Make the Tonic Combo: Boil 1 pint of water. Add 2 teaspoons dried, cut pseudoginseng root. Cover, simmer for 5 minutes, and then set aside. Steep 10 minutes. Uncover and add the scraped pollen from 1 cattail. Stir thoroughly, replace the lid, and steep another 10 minutes. Strain and drink COOL, *never* warm.

DYSMENORRHEA

(see Cramps and Menstrual Difficulties)

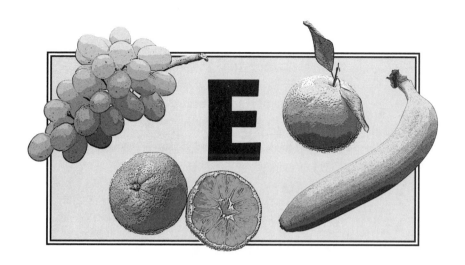

ECZEMA

Cold Black Tea Good for Red, Itchy Skin

DESCRIPTION

Eczema (also called dermatitis) is a common skin inflammation. The problem is manifested with the appearance of red, raised lesions that are weeping and, in the acute stage, crusted. In the chronic stage eczema is marked by scaly, red, thickened patches of skin, often attributed to rubbing or scratching. Ordinarily this doesn't pose a serious health risk and is easily treated with herbal liquids and salves.

Retired Dermatologist Likes His Cup of Tea on the Skin Instead of Inside His System

For 37 years, Nelson Radcliffe, M.D., practiced his specialty of medicine, dermatology, before retiring in 1973. When we met about 15 years later at a national health convention held in Cleveland, Ohio, we exchanged information about the care of the skin. He had accompanied his wife to my lecture on "Folk Remedies from Around the World." He was intrigued with what I had to say about tea in general.

He shared with me something I had never heard of before. Dr. Radcliffe said that in his practice he often relied upon *cold* black tea to help his patients suffering from eczema. He would recommend that they make a *strong* tea and bathe the skin with it four or five times each day. Invariably the itchiness and redness would disappear in a few days after successive treatments.

ANTI-ITCH TEA

1 pint spring or distilled water
10 black-tea bags

Boil the water; add the tea bags; cover, set aside and steep 30 minutes. DO NOT strain; refrigerate with tea bags intact. Bathe skin as recommended.

EDEMA

Getting Rid of Excess Fluid with More Fluid

DESCRIPTION

In order to make richly flavored iced tea, you need to begin by using high-quality herbs. Remember, you get what you pay for: cheap herbs equal unpleasant tea, whereas good herbs yield flavorful tea. The kind to look for are those with a strong aroma and bright color; they usually have the best flavor, too.

Although I've given a number of different ways so far in this text as to how teas can be made, I haven't mentioned this method yet. In some ways (at least for making iced tea) it is preferable to others that have already been suggested. I advise that iced teas be brewed in jars with lids, which keep the aromatic substances—the parts that taste best—from escaping.

Quart canning jars are the most suitable for this, because they seal tightly and are made from heat-resistant glass. Place the herbs in the bottom of the jar, pour boiling water over them to fill the jar, then put the lid on tightly. Let them cool for an hour, then strain and add honey if you like. Add water to bring the volume back to a quart again, if necessary.

Iced Teas that Help You Lose Those Liquid Pounds

Abnormally large amounts of fluid in the intercellular tissue spaces of the body can be due to venous or lymphatic obstruction, to increased vascular permeability, or due to heart failure or kidney disease. The best way, believe it or not, to remove such excess fluid is by putting *more* fluid into the body. As strange as this seems, it really *does* work.

Over the years I've experimented with a number of different herbs that are quite useful in treating edema. Most of these have been taken in the form of capsules or *warm* herbal teas. But I became really excited one time in my research upon discovering just how well *iced* teas worked for this same problem; in fact, they work *better* than hot teas do. By what mechanism this is done, however, remains to be found.

The following two recipes are wonderful for edema. They should be drunk on a daily basis with and without meals.

VIVID HERBAL COOLER

It is pretty well known by now that rose hips are rich in vitamin C and yield a delicious, light, fruity flavor when cooked. Spearmint, on the other hand, has a cooling and refreshing quality to it. When they are combined to make iced tea they form a delightful tonic the body loves.

> *12 tbsp. rose hips*
>
> *6 tbsp. spearmint*
>
> *1 1/4 quarts mineral or seltzer water*
>
> *juice of 2 limes*

Mix together the rose hips and spearmint; brew as directed under the Description subheading. Add lime juice after the tea has been refrigerated.

HERBAL GINGER BEER

Ginger root contains an oily resin called gingerol, which is very helpful in treating indigestion, muscle inflammation and pain, arthritis, and migraine headaches.

> *1 inch piece of ginger root, peeled and chopped*
>
> *1 1/4 quarts of spring or distilled water*
>
> *juice of two lemons*
>
> *blackstrap molasses for sweetening to taste*

Simmer the ginger root in water, covered, over low heat for 25 minutes. Strain, adding more water as needed. Cool slightly for about 10 minutes. Then add the lemon juice and molasses. The tea should still be warm enough to dissolve the molasses or the molasses may collect on the bottom of the container.

EMPHYSEMA

Utah Cattle Rancher Treats Lung Condition with Herbal Tea

DESCRIPTION

Emphysema is a lung condition characterized by an abnormal increase in the size of air spaces distal to the terminal bronchiole, which are those parts containing alveoli; when this disease is present there are destructive changes in the walls of the alveoli and reduction in their number.

Emphysema is marked by minimal coughing, scant sputum, shortness of breath, weight loss, infections, barrel chest, minimal wheezing, pursed-lip breathing, slight bluish discoloration of the skin and mucous membranes, and very diminished breathing sounds.

"First the Elk Story, Then the Remedy"

Cyrus Johnson has been a rancher for 55 years of his life. "I'm pushing 79 pretty soon," he drawled, "and all I know is cows and alfalfa." Then with a wink, he slyly added, "'Course I might know a thing or two 'bout horses and gardening."

I met him awhile back during a cattle auction sale going on in Southern Utah. He was these selling some feeder calves and a couple of bulls, and I was there to bid and buy. As the day proceeded and we got to know each other a little better, I inquired if he knew any folk remedies that might have been handed down through his family.

He replied, "Yep, I know one. It's a sure-fire remedy that has kept me breathing for many years, otherwise I'd probably be dead by now." He said he had been troubled with emphysema for years, but finally gave one of his grandma's old remedies a try. "It sure worked out good for me," he admitted with pride. "I can honestly say that our grandparents knew a lot more 'bout doctoring than we do."

I eagerly pressed him for the remedy. He responded this way: "I'll tell you what you want to know, but only on one condition." I steeled my nerves not knowing exactly what to expect, but prepared for outlandish terms, nevertheless. I was dumbfounded when he stated what he wanted.

155

"I'm going to tell you a true elk-hunting story *before* I give you my 'secret' family remedy," he said with a chuckle. "You'll not only have to listen to it, but you'll have to agree to put it in this here book you say you're going to be writing soon. That's the agreement!"

I said I had no problems with that and we shook hands on the matter. "Now for my story," he said.

Elk Hunter Shoots Horse on Purpose

During the October 1995 elk hunt on Boulder Mountain (in southwestern Utah), my informant began, two men from out of state by the names of Davis and Pierce camped together at Haws Pasture, just five miles northwest of Boulder on Bear Creek. Both men had taken a week off for the hunt. But upon returning to their camp on a Saturday, they found that a tire on the Davis truck had been severely slashed with a strong knife. The next day they left camp to look for more elk and returned that evening to find that two more truck tires had been deliberately slashed.

After spending much of their Sunday traveling to Escalante and Boulder for tire and tube repairs, the two hunters devised a scheme where on the following Monday Davis would stake out their camp and Pierce would hunt nearby in case the mysterious slasher might return. Neither man could conceive, though, why on earth anyone would want to slash their tires so far out in the wilderness, away from gangs and criminal elements.

Around 9 A.M. on Monday, Davis pulled his high-powered gun scope from his rifle and watched through it some distance away, being well hidden in the trees. Soon another hunter named Button from Kanab, Utah, rode up on his thoroughbred quarter horse. He looked around leisurely and then slowly dismounted and went directly over to Davis's truck. He again carefully surveyed the area to make sure no one was in sight. He then went to the back part of the vehicle and stood there for a moment.

Davis watched in utter amazement through his scope as Button withdrew a large pearl-handled Bowie knife from the leather sheath he wore on his belt and proceeded to make a number of vicious stabbing cuts in the left rear tire. After doing this, the man quickly headed for his horse. Not wanting the vandal to get away from him, Davis immediately picked up his rifle and shot the other man's horse between the eyes.

His hunting partner Pierce, upon hearing the nearby shot, quickly ran back to camp. Both men placed Button under citizens' arrest and transported him in Pierce's truck down to the convenience store in Boulder to call local authorities.

The deputy sheriff of Garfield County, a fellow by the name of Luker, came out later that morning and listened to both sides of this bizarre affair. Button denied having slashed any tires. And since only Davis had seen the act and not his friend Pierce, it was only one man's word against that of another. When Luker asked Button why he was in the Davis camp, the guy replied that he and Davis had been chasing the same elk earlier in the hunt and he (Button) just wanted to see if the other men had gotten the elk or not.

Button claimed he was out a $3,000 horse, and the two out-of-state hunters told Luker they were out about $700 in tires and had lost several valuable days of their expensive vacation and hunting trip. The deputy sheriff advised all three men to "stop acting like a bunch of spoiled kids" and to try and work out their differences between them "like real men do." He advised them to "call it a draw" and to go their separate ways.

The peace officer drove Button back up the mountain to his truck and empty horse trailer, just to make certain the parties did-n't tangle with each other any more. Davis and Pierce decided to call it quits and head back home four days early. In Boulder they met my rancher informant and subsequently told him of the whole affair. They called this experience "the hunting trip from Hell" and vowed never to come back to that part of Utah to hunt elk. Pierce even grumbled that he might become a vegetarian after this wacky ordeal.

"Are You Ready to Hear My Remedy?"

Mr. Johnson finished his tale and then asked me, "Are your ready now to hear my remedy?" I nodded in the affirmative and he continued speaking.

He started telling me about Brigham or Mormon tea, assuming I had never heard of it before. And when I spoke up saying that I already knew about it, he stated "Don't interrupt me; let me tell it my way, okay?" I remained silent after that, jotting down the highlights of what he had to say in a little spiral notebook I carry with me at all times in one of the pockets of my cotton shirts.

This herb has already been mentioned at some length under DYSENTERY. But Johnson's use of it for this particular lung ailment was original, to say the least. He described how he makes a tea every morning and drinks 2 or 3 cups throughout the day "whenever I feel my breathing is becoming difficult again," he said. "Sometimes I'll even mix a little dried peppermint in with these shrub stems: it makes for one heckuva delicious tea, not to mention making my lungs fine."

CYRUS' EMPHYSEMA TEA

1¹/₂ pints boiling water

2 tbsp. Brigham or Mormon tea (Ephedra species)

1 tbsp. dried peppermint leaves

Add the Brigham tea first; cover and simmer on low heat a few minutes. Then remove lid and add the mint leaves. Stir and replace lid. Set aside to steep for 30 minutes. Strain only one cup at a time. Reheat to lukewarm before drinking. Drink throughout the day until tea is gone. Make a fresh batch each day; don't refrigerate overnight.

ENDOMETRIOSIS

Genetic Research Assistant Uses Alfalfa and Red Clover Teas to Prevent "Career Woman's Disease"

DESCRIPTION

Endometriosis has been classified by at least one female medical doctor as being "the illness of competition." In her outstanding book, *Women's Bodies, Women's Wisdom* (New York: Bantam Books, 1994, p. 138) Christiane Northrup, M.D., writes that endometriosis "comes about when a woman's emotional needs are competing with her functioning in the outside world." The author states that every time a working woman's innermost emotional needs get in direct conflict with what her surrounding job and home environments demand of her, then "endometriosis is one of the ways in which her body tries to draw her attention to the problem." Dr. Northrup goes on to point out that "a great many of the women I've seen who have endometriosis drive themselves relentlessly in the outer world, rarely resting, rarely tuning in to their innermost needs and deepest desires." So, she reasons, "it makes perfect sense that so many women would have this disease" at this time in our nation's history. "It is," Dr. Northrup believes, "our bodies trying not to let us forget our feminine nature, our need for self-nurturance, and our connection with other women."

The Mouse with a Human Ear on Its Back

The woman whom I'm indebted to for the two tea remedies mentioned in this section is quite normal, although one may wonder if some of the work she's involved with isn't just a tad like something from a carnival sideshow perhaps. I'm referring, of course, to Kay (she didn't want her real name to be used with this story). Kay works in research laboratories in Boston.

She has been involved for some time with a type of science considered to be on the leading edge of technological research; it is known as tissue engineering, which permits labs to grow skin and cartilage for transplant in humans.

A specially bred species of mice lacking immune systems are vital to the process. Kay works on a research team consisting of plastic surgeons, anesthesiologists, and chemical engineers. They had been asked by surgeons from Children's Hospital in Boston to come up with a suitable replacement for children born without ears or for young kids who've accidentally had one of their ears chewed off by a dog.

So her team set about creating an earlike scaffolding, she said, of porous, biodegradable polyester fiber. Then they distributed human cartilage cells throughout the form and implanted the prototype ear on the back of a hairless mouse.

Because the rodent had no immune system, its body didn't reject the human tissue. In fact, the ear was slowly nourished on the animal's back as the cartilage cells grew to replace the fiber. Once they surgically removed the ear, the mouse remained healthy and alive.

"We ended up with a piece of cartilage in the shape of an ear," she said over the phone. But this is "just the beginning," she insisted. "We've already managed to grow liver, skin, cartilage, bone, ureters, heart valves, tendons, intestines, blood vessels, and breast tissue on such polymer scaffolding."

I couldn't resist ribbing her a little bit during our conversation. At one point, I asked in mocked innocence, "Who did you say was the principal doctor you worked with in this research? Wasn't it Dr. Frankenstein, I believe?" She enjoyed the good humor at her expense without getting offended.

"So, tell me about the teas you've been using to help alleviate some of your pelvic pain, abnormal menstrual cycles, and infertility," I said.

Kay said that she has been "one of those health food nuts you hear about so much" for quite some time now. "Once when I went to a Bread & Circus up here," she continued, "I met this clerk who was pretty knowledgeable about herbs. The lady recommended alfalfa and red clover for me after hearing about my problem." (Bread & Circus is a small chain of very large health food supermarkets in the greater Boston area.)

Kay tried the herbs by capsule for about a month, but nothing seemed to work for her. So she decided to buy the dried, cut forms of the herbs and make teas out of them. "That's when I started getting some results," she mentioned. "But it was too much of a hassle making two teas, so I finally settled for a blend of both, which seems to have worked well for me."

She drinks three to four cups of the blend each day and claims to have experienced no further pain. Also, her menses is fairly regular now, and she noted, "I'm expecting my first child next May (1996) sometime."

Her last comments again had to do with the project of growing replacement parts for humans on animals. "Right now we have some pretty amazing skin products that are in the advanced stages of clinical testing on humans," she observed. "And we have heart valves just entering the first phase of clinical trials, but I can't really talk too much about them right now, or else I might lose my job. That's pretty hush-hush stuff around here.

"But someday," she said with enthusiasm in her voice, "we'll be able to grow ears and noses right inside a test tube using a patient's own cells on a custom-designed scaffold. And other tissues can be grown from donated cells on similar polymer devices placed in the patient's own body." She predicted that the next major advances to come in the field of reconstructive surgery would be from tissue engineering.

Still, I think, as broad-minded and liberal as I am, that there are certain boundaries humans were never intended to cross in their experiments with the processes of life itself. How this may be regarded by Heaven is probably best left up to theologians. But I, for one, think it doesn't bode too well with the Creator Himself.

HORMONE TEA

The most common therapy for endometriosis, once it has been properly diagnosed by a qualified doctor, is hormonal therapy. Kay discovered several natural sources of hormones, thanks to the female clerk at one of the Bread & Circus stores. Here is Kay's own special formula blend.

> **5 cups boiling water**
>
> **1 tbsp. alfalfa leaves**
>
> **1 tbsp. red clover blossoms**
>
> **wild honey to sweeten**

After the water starts boiling, add both herbs. Stir with a spoon, cover the pot with a lid, and set aside to steep for about 15 minutes. Strain and drink one cup while still quite warm. Add a little honey to improve the taste, if necessary. Drink with every meal. Continue this pattern of consumption for up to six months or more, as needed.

The *Encyclopedia of Common Natural Ingredients Used in Food, Drugs and Cosmetics* by Albert Leung (New York: John Wiley & Sons, 1980, pp. 15; 132–133) has been a standard desk reference for scientists such as myself for a number of years. It mentions that alfalfa is rich in hormonelike compounds such as coumestrol, medicagol, genistein, biochanin A, and daidzein, while clover tops have more of the same things.

EPILEPSY

Naturopathic Tonic Reduces the Incidence of Seizures

DESCRIPTION

Epilepsy can be any of a group of syndromes characterized by paroxysmal passing disturbances of brain function. These may be manifested either as episodes of memory loss or unconsciousness, abnormal muscle function, psychic or sensory disturbances, or upset of the autonomic nervous system.

A single episode is termed a seizure. Different kinds of epilepsy are nothing more than combinations of various types of seizures. Symptoms are due to paroxysmal disturbance of the electrical activity of the brain.

Nation's First Government-Run Natural Medical Clinic

The King County Council of Washington State (which includes the capital of Seattle) recently recommended to federal health officials that Bastyr University be seriously considered for operating the nation's first government-run alternative medicine clinic.

Bastyr University is America's largest and only fully accredited, multidisciplinary naturopathic medicine college. It originated from humble beginnings many years ago in Seattle. The current president, Joe Pizzorno, N.D., is himself a practitioner and teacher of natural medicine. He has been the main inspiration behind this very innovative concept.

His clear intention for this first-ever public health clinic using only natural remedies is to see if such a facility will meet the public's needs and to determine if the results are as good as or better than conventional medical treatment. Pizzorno noted in an interview that there are many cases of alternative practitioners and regular medical doctors working together in practices nationwide. But the key element in something like this, he observed, is getting government services to offer natural-remedy options to their huge clientele. The only reason federal agencies might ever consider doing that is if they can somehow save money in the process. Dr. Pizzorno thought that the cost-effectiveness of natural remedies had opened many doors for an educational institution such as the one he currently presides over.

"In a number of health situations," he emphasized, "natural therapies are more appropriate and less expensive in the long run because they address prevention and lifestyle modification. By moving natural medicine into our health care system, we can eliminate some of the problems currently challenging that system—which isn't truly health care but rather disease treatment."

Kent Pullen, the chairperson of the King County Council, fully concurred with Pizzorno's views. "More often than not," he told this author by telephone, "orthodox medicine focuses solely on the symptoms of the problem and seldom ever actually deals with the root cause of it. Either a prescription drug is written to help dull the patient's pain, or an operation is recommended to remove a diseased organ. The real cause of sickness hasn't yet been fully investigated. That's why I and the rest of the city county council members wanted to take a natural approach with this clinic and avail the people of vitamins, minerals, enzymes, herbs, and other natural healing modalities that can assist the body in healing itself better. Natural remedies aren't just more effective, but they have fewer side effects and are usually less expensive because of their preventative aspects."

The King County Council is the twelfth largest county-governing body in the United States. Pullen and a dozen other members (about two thirds of the council) have used natural remedies in some form for a number of years. Besides this unified health philosophy, they also were anxious to see alternative medicine covered by insurance companies.

With the help of such an open-minded and willing group, Pizzorno and other natural medicine practitioners in the state were able to persuade *all* council members to recommend to U.S. government officials that Bastyr University be chosen for managing the country's first federal-run natural remedies public health clinic.

Epilepsy Diminished with Homeopathic Tonic

One of the members of the King County Council with whom I spoke by phone became an advocate of natural remedies when a naturopathic physician at Bastyr University was able to successfully treat the individual's 17-year-old daughter's epilepsy. This person, however, asked that I not mention any name, age, occupation, or sexual gender; hence, I will, hereafter, only refer to my informant as Person X.

"I took her to a number of regular medical specialists, all of whom prescribed many different kinds of medications for her. But none seemed to help her as much as the few simple remedies that a doctor from over at the school [Bastyr University] recommended for her." My informant then read to me over the line the various things that the girl had been taking for about eight months, with apparently very good results. "At first I was giving her these liquid medicines orally [beneath the tongue], but after awhile decided to put them in some kind of juice, which she liked better." Person X claimed that this innovative tonic "really helped my girl a lot," in that the number of seizures she routinely experienced were diminished by about 70 percent. "Instead of her having two or three seizures a week as before," Person X stated, "she now gets by with only *one* every six weeks or two months."

These particular remedies may be obtained from some health food stores or by mail from one of the following trio of pharmaceutical suppliers who sell homeopathic drugs:

Boericke & Tafel, Inc.
1011 Arch St.
Philadelphia, PA 19107

Horton & Converse
621 W. Pico Blvd.
Los Angeles, CA 90015

Kiehl Pharmacy, Inc.
109 Third Avenue
New York, NY 10003

The juice Person X later employed as the medium by which these natural medicines were carried into her daughter's system was chlorophyll. This she purchased directly from Pines International of Lawrence, Kansas (see Product Appendix), and mixed with spring or distilled water. The complete tonic itself is given below.

ANTI-SEIZURE TONIC MEDICINE

Sulfur 5M (flowers of sulfur: concentration of 1:5000)

Calcarea (Calcarea ostrearum or calcium carbonate from oyster shells)

Lycopodium (Lycopodium clavatum or club moss)

1 8-oz. glass of water

1 tsp. Pines wheat grass juice concentrate powder

$1/_2$ tsp. Pines barley juice concentrate powder

Mix the last three ingredients together first. Stir the cereal grass powders so they are thoroughly dissolved in the water (use only spring or distilled for this, never from the tap).

Then add the first three ingredients in the exact order given, according to the suggested amounts indicated on the package or container labels. Stir in well before drinking.

In the beginning, it may be necessary for the epileptic client to drink two glasses of this tonic each day for several months at a time. But as the severity of the problem is allayed, it may be necessary to take only one glass of it every other day or twice weekly.

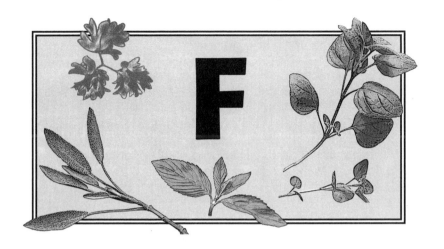

FALSE LABOR

An Herbal Tea Preventive

DESCRIPTION

Labor is defined by doctors as being that function of the female organism by which the product of conception is finally expelled from the uterus through the vagina to the outside world.

False labor (also called mimetic labor or false pains) are ineffective rhythmic pains that resemble the real thing but that are not accompanied by effacement and dilation of the cervix. In *The Motherhood Report,* authors Eva Margolies and Louis Genevie, Ph.D., noted that some women are more apt to experience false labor than are others:

- ▌ Women who experience more cramping during their periods seem to be more susceptible to false labor pains.

- ▌ Women of lower socioeconomic status and with less education tend to report more false pains.

- ▌ Younger mothers are apt to have more false labors than older mothers do.

- ▌ Researchers have found that first-time mothers usually experience more anxiety along with increased incidents of false labor than do second-time moms.

Appalachian Mountain Folk Remedy

The Appalachians are an extensive mountain system running in a broad belt for about 1,600 miles southwest from the Gaspé Peninsula in Quebec province, Canada, to the Gulf coastal plain in Alabama. Main sections in the system are the White Mountains, Green Mountains, Berkshire Hills, Catskill Mountains, the Allegheny Plateau, Black Mountains, Great Smoky Mountains, the Blue Ridge Mountains, and the Cumberland Plateau.

Down in the south where the Appalachian Mountains run through Alabama, folk medicine among the common people is alive and well. I interviewed several herbalists some years back regarding their use of birthroot for labor problems. They said the plant's foul odor reminded them a lot of the stench of rotting flesh, and for this reason they often make an ointment from the rhizomes and roots for treating gangrene.

They claim that when a woman drinks some of the root tea, her false pains soon cease without inducing real labor too early in the pregnancy. Here is the method most often used in the preparation of this fine remedy.

TEA FOR FALSE PAINS

1 pint water

2 tsp. coarsely chopped, fresh or dried birthroot

Boil the water. Then add the birthroot, cover with lid, and simmer on low heat for 6 minutes. Set aside and steep for 15 minutes. Strain and drink one cup of *warm* tea twice daily on an empty stomach or whenever false pains occur.

FIBROADENOMA

Chlorophyll and Beet Juice Should Keep a Benign Tumor from Becoming Malignant

DESCRIPTION

A fibroadenoma has been defined by one doctor as being a benign or nonmalignant tumor that most commonly occurs in young women who are 20 or 30 something. Such a growth can be between one to two inches in size and is believed to form by the growth of connective tissue in the lobules. A tumor of this kind is usually firm and smooth and is seldom found in older women.

Fibroadenomas can develop rapidly when they are stimulated by the increased hormones of pregnancy or by oral contraceptives and, with age, they may harden and change into calcium. In approximately 85 percent of cases, only one fibroadenoma will be present in a woman's breast; but if a woman does develop one, she has about a 15 percent chance of getting a second tumor some years later.

A few published medical studies of late have attempted to demonstrate a relationship between fibroadenomas and a woman's risk of eventually developing breast cancer sometime in her life. But while there is a slight chance of this happening, it still doesn't mean surgeons need to remove this mass if it has been properly diagnosed as being a fibroadenoma.

Prevention Treatment

Technically speaking, once a woman develops a nonmalignant tumor of this kind there is very little she can do to get rid of it through natural remedies; surgery remains about the only elective option for those women who don't like the idea of living with a palpable mass in their breasts.

There is, however, a simple juice combination that may be of considerable help for younger women in preventing the development of fibroadenomas. It is a blend of chlorophyll and beet juice taken on a regular basis with meals. Those women in their twenties or thirties who have relied on this tonic for several years and have been properly examined by qualified doctors showed *no* incidence of fibroadenoma development.

Juice Tonic for Healthy Breasts

It is much easier to make this simple combination by using *powdered* juice concentrates instead of making it from scratch, which can take time that you may not always have.

> *1 tsp. Pines barley juice concentrate*
>
> *1 tsp. Pines wheat grass juice concentrate*
>
> *1 tsp. Pines beet juice concentrate*
>
> *1 tsp. liquid Kyolic Garlic*
>
> *1$^1/_2$ glasses or 12 fluid ounces cool spring or distilled water*

Mix the powdered ingredients in with the suggested amount of water. This can be done by stirring everything thoroughly with a spoon for several minutes by pouring the water followed by the dried juice powders into a Vita-Mix whole food machine, adding three ice cubes, securing the two-part lid in place, and then mixing the contents for one minute. Divide into equal parts and drink twice daily with meals.

(See the Product Appendix under Pines, Kyolic, and Vita-Mix for more information on obtaining any of these fine items. A new health drink from Pines called Mighty Green can be substituted for the barley juice and wheat juice concentrate, if desired.)

FIBROCYSTIC DISEASE

Correct Information, Not Remedies,
Is What Is Needed Here

DESCRIPTION

This is probably the only entry in the entire book that will *not* list any specific remedies. The reason for this is quite simple: "Fibrocystic disease" isn't really a disease after all. In fact, it may more accurately be termed "medical mislabeling" by the very health care profession to which millions of women have looked and trusted for presumably reliable information.

Two medical books devoted exclusively to women's health issues and written by competent doctors who are well-qualified to discuss such matters both take issue with "fibrocystic disease." The authors of both works are in general agreement that most women have virtually *nothing to worry about* if they've been previously told by some health care provider that they have such a problem.

Christiane Northrup, M.D. has been a practicing physician using natural methods for well over a decade. She has been past president of the American Holistic Medical Association and a founding partner in a women's health clinic in Yarmouth, Maine. She wrote *Women's Bodies, Women's Wisdom* (New York: Bantam, 1994). She said that a major medical study done of this problem in 1985 determined that a full 80 percent of what had been previously called fibrocystic disease was "actually normal changes in breast anatomy" and had *no* association whatsoever with an increase in breast cancer (as many doctors had erroneously informed their patients was the case).

John Davidson, M.D., has been in practice for over a quarter of a century as a general and vascular surgeon. For the last 15 years he has been practicing medicine at North Dallas's Presbyterian Hospital, where over 50 percent of his patients are women with breast problems. He is considered to be one of the country's top experts in breast health. He co-authored the book *In Touch with Your Breasts: The Answers to Women's Questions On Breastcare* (Waco, TX: WRS Publishing, 1995) with freelance health writer Jan Winebrenner. He made very plain that "the term fibrocystic disease is inaccurate" because it is a "normal breast condition [and] not a disease."

Both doctors pointed out that normal fibrocystic *changes* do occur in breast tissue with each menstrual cycle and that such changes also accompany the natural aging process. Breasts are made up of fat and connective tissue. But as the female body slowly ages, the ratio of connective tissue to fat changes considerably. Breast glandular cells and ductal cells die and are replaced with either fibrous tissue or with fat tissue. Therefore, one area of the breast might be denser than another simply because there is likely to be more fat tissue in that area than in another place. This replacement of the breast tissue in uneven distributions causes the breast to become more lumpy than usual. But women shouldn't panic when pathologists turn up very high fibrocystic changes in their breast biopsies; it is perfectly normal and usually nothing to fret over.

FIBROID TUMORS

(see Fiboradenoma)

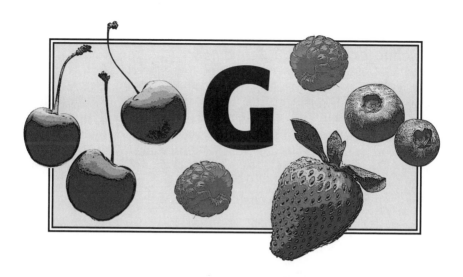

GALACTORRHEA

Green Tea–Rasberry Leaf Fruit Drink Stops Unnecessary Milk Production

DESCRIPTION

Galactorrhea is a condition in which a woman's breasts tend to secrete a milky-white substance when there is no need for it. Close to 40 percent of such cases result from unknown causes, but the remainder of them are usually associated with amenorrhea (see under the alphabetized entries for more on this) or with ovulatory dysfunction.

In other instances the problem may be induced by prescription drugs, especially those medications that cause the pituitary gland to generate inappropriate secretions of prolactin (lactating hormone from the anterior pituitary). In those cases where such a thing may occur due to elevated prolactin, a doctor might want to submit his female patient to a CT scan of the brain to determine if there is a tumor on the pituitary itself. If no tumor or other causes are found for severe galactorrhea, then a woman may find relief in drinking herbal teas high in tannic acid. These include bayberry bark, blackberry bark, black tea, lemon balm, and Chinese turkey rhubarb root. Tannins seem to be the key here in controlling excess prolactin production. Instructions for making them appear at the end of this entry.

Delightful Tea Drink Halts Breast Milk

Some women who have opted for natural remedies to treat their galactorrhea have reported to me several different tea or fruit drinks that have helped to reduce their breast milklike secretions. The Anthropological Research Center in Salt Lake City (of which I've been the director for the past 19 years) combined all these ingredients together in one formula and tested it on female volunteers suffering from this problem. Eleven of the 17 of them reported immediate results within 48 hours after taking three to five glasses of this delicious herb-tea–fruit drink.

PREPARATION OF TEA-FRUIT DRINK

1$^1/_4$ cups iced green tea

1 cup cold raspberry leaf tea

1 cup fresh or unsweetened frozen raspberries

$^1/_2$ cup fresh pineapple chunks

1 kiwi fruit, peeled

$^1/_2$ large pear, unpeeled

1 cup ice cubes

To make iced teas, place three green tea bags in one empty pint jar and one tablespoon raspberry leaves in another glass jar. Then pour 1$^1/_2$ cups boiling water over each of them. Screw the lids on tightly and let them cool for an hour, then strain and refrigerate in separate clean containers. Then pour them into a Vita-Mix Total Nutrition Center and add the rest of the ingredients in the order given. Secure the two-part lid in place and blend for 2 minutes. Divide into three equal portions and refrigerate; drink one part every 12 to 16 hours for two days. If necessary, this amount can be doubled and taken every eight hours within the same time period.

Making Other Teas

When excess prolactin secretion is suspected as being the primary cause of galactorrhea, teas known for their high tannin contents may be of considerable value in alleviating this problem. Teas recommended for this include roots (rhubarb), barks (bayberry and blackberry), and herbs (black tea and lemon balm).

They are prepared in separate ways. Because roots and barks are made of tougher material, they require more cooking.

First Method: Boil one pint of water. Add 1¹/₂ tablespoons of rhubarb OR bayberry OR blackberry. (Be sure to make each of these *separately;* DO NOT mix together in one pot.) Cover with a lid, lower heat, and simmer for 5 minutes. Set aside and steep for 35 minutes. Strain and store in clean containers in the refrigerator. Drink one cup twice daily with meals.

Second Method: Boil one pint of water. Set aside and add either four teabags OR one tablespoon of black tea OR lemon balm. (Make each of these teas in separate pots.) Cover with a lid and steep for 35 minutes. Strain and refrigerate. Drink two cups each day on an empty stomach.

GALLBLADDER PROBLEMS

Fruit, Vegetable, and Herb Therapies for the Gallbladder

DESCRIPTION

For many people the gallbladder is one of those organs of the body that they seem to know very little about. In order to help those who may be unfamiliar with it, here is a little information for them.

The gallbladder is a small, pear-shaped organ located immediately below the liver. Its primary functions are to concentrate and store bile (a substance produced by the liver to aid in the emulsification [digestion] of fats). Bile is stored in the gallbladder and judiciously secreted during digestion into the duodenum, the portion of the small intestine joined to the stomach.

The formation of gallstones (called cholelithiasis in medical terms) is the most common problem for this organ. It generally occurs when excessive amounts of cholesterol in the bile clump together in solid masses. The quantity and size of gallstones may vary from one large stone or several medium-sized ones to hundreds of tiny ones no bigger than pea gravel. There are "silent" stones that cause no pain and need no treatment to aggressive gallstones that can block the bile duct or cause inflammation, thereby producing a great deal of pain and misery.

In some instances an infected gallbladder may become filled with purulent matter (a medical condition called empyema). Gallstones occur more frequently in women than in men.

Dealing with the Pain

One thing I learned many years ago when beginning in this business of helping people across America find simple solutions to complex health problems is that those experiencing great suffering want something first of all to relieve their excruciating pains. They don't care for theories or philosophies; they want just a short explanation of what can be taken to help ease their physical agonies.

So it is then with gallstones that I wish to recommend the consumption of *warm* catnip tea throughout the day. Having suggested this to hundreds of individuals in the last couple of decades and having been a personal witness to just how well it has worked for so many, I dare to venture this humble guarantee: If 1 to 2 cups of *warm* catnip tea fail to relieve the pain of a gallstone moving around inside someone's system, then that individual can write me personally, and I will gladly report the entire contents of said letter in my next health book. *That* is how sure I am of this remedy.

CATNIP PAIN RELIEVER

2$^1/_2$ cups boiling water
1$^1/_4$ level tbsp. dried, cut catnip herb

Add the herb to the water. Stir with a spoon. Cover with lid and set aside to steep for 25 minutes. Strain and drink 1–2 cups of *warm* tea on an *empty* stomach to stop the pain; the effect usually lasts for several hours. Repeat as often as necessary.

Getting Rid of Gallstones

One of the most effective treatments for expelling gallstones from the system calls for the use of olive oil and a combination of grapefruit juice and apple cider vinegar in water, to be taken over a period of several days or weeks, if necessary.

However, this therapy works only on an empty stomach and should be taken first thing in the morning and again in the evening around 7 P.M.

STEP ONE: Take two tablespoons of olive oil before breakfast.

STEP TWO: Mix together $^1/_2$ cup pink or white grapefruit juice, 1 tablespoon apple cider vinegar, and $^1/_4$ cup spring or distilled water.

STEP THREE: Drink immediately after taking the olive oil.

STEP FOUR: Repeat same procedures again at night. Do this for 5, 10, or 15 days.

STEP FIVE: Lie down on your right side for several hours after doing this, if possible. Put a pillow under the right side of your rib cage, so that the gallbladder is in a sloping position to better enable the stones to slip out and be more easily eliminated in the next few bowel movements.

Treating an Infected Gallbladder

Two of the best nutrients for combating infection in the gallbladder are vitamins A and C. But instead of simply taking tablets or capsules, I advise a person to drink vegetable juices rich in both nutrients.

ANTI-INFECTION JUICE

¹/₂ cup carrot juice (canned)

¹/₂ cup spinach juice (canned)

¹/₂ cup V-8 juice (low-sodium and canned)

1 tbsp. Pines beet juice concentrate powder

1 tsp. Pines rhubarb juice concentrate powder

Mix everything together in the order given in a Vita-Mix Total Nutrition Center or equivalent food blender. Make sure the top lid is properly secured in place so that no mess results when the unit is turned on. Mix for about 1¹/₂ minutes. Drink at least once each day with a meal.

Reducing Bladder Inflammation

Two remedies are handy for reducing inflammation of the gallbladder. One is pear juice: Drink at least two cups every day. To make pear juice, combine 3 pear halves in a food blender with one cup of spring or distilled water.

If a person has blood sugar problems (such as diabetes or hypoglycemia), however, which preclude the use of any sweet fruits such as pears, then a tea made from marshmallow roots is helpful instead. Boil two cups of water, then add 1¹/₂ tablespoons of dried, cut marshmallow root. Stir, cover with a lid, reduce heat, and simmer for 7 minutes. Set aside and steep another 15 minutes. Strain, and drink *warm* on an empty stomach.

GLAUCOMA

What Some Doctors in Rome Have Done for This Eye Problem

DESCRIPTION

Glaucoma is a disorder characterized by an increase in intraocular pressure, that is to say, a build-up of pressure within the eyeball. A clear fluid inside the eyeball called aqueous humor provides nutrients to and carries away waste products from the lens and cornea of the eye. Each day, the eye produces about one teaspoon of this special eye fluid. Ordinarily, this liquid escapes from the eye through a spongy mesh of connective tissue at about the same rate at which it is produced. But in glaucoma, production of this fluid exceeds the rate of its escape.

Do Italian Ophthalmologists Have Something Better for This Problem?

While there is certainly no proven way to actually prevent glaucoma from occurring, early detection and self-treatment could prevent damage to the optic nerve. A qualified ophthalmologist should conduct an eye exam every two years on those over the age of 50. But those who are African-Americans should start seeing an eye doctor beginning at the age of 38.

Some years ago I happened to spend a few days in Rome and had a chance to interview some doctors there who where using natural remedies in a portion of their medical practices. A few of them were ophthalmologists, and they relied heavily on the herbal extract of bilberry for helping many of their older patients suffering from a variety of eye disorders: glaucoma, diabetic retinopathy, retinitis pigmentosa, macular degeneration, hemorrhagic retinopathy, night and day blindness, and nearsightedness.

Today bilberry is widely available in most health food stores, nutrition centers, and herb shops. It is sold in fluid extract, capsule, and tea forms. The Italian doctors with whom I spoke had always recommended bilberry *tea* as the most ideal form in which to take this herb for the best results possible.

BILBERRY TONIC FOR HEALTHY EYES

2 1/2 cups distilled water
1 1/4 tbsp. dried bilberries
3/4 tbsp. dried, cut bilberry leaves

Boil the water, then add the berries. Cover with a lid, lower heat, and simmer 4 minutes. Remove the lid and add the leaves. Stir thoroughly and replace the lid. Set aside and steep for 20 minutes. Strain and drink one cup twice daily on an empty stomach.

My Italian informants also speculated that glaucoma might even be considered to be a type of "stress-induced" eye problem. In their many years of evaluating thousands of patients with many different types of eye disorders, they discovered, quite by accident, that those who were "hot tempered" or "easily argumentative" were most likely to have *higher* incidence of glaucoma than those who were more even tempered and had mellow personalities. The "secret" here (if it can truly be called that) seems to be that *less* mental and emotional stress could possibly prevent or, at the very least, reduce the risks of incurring this particular eye disorder.

These Italian doctors also mentioned that those who regularly consumed citrus fruits (or their juices) had *less* incidence of glaucoma or *reduced* symptoms of it.

GOUT

An Old Russian Cossack Remedy for Uric Acid Accumulations

Description

Gout is a disorder affecting *all* the major and minor organs of the body. It is usually manifested by sudden and severe joint pain (particularly in the big toe), swelling and redness around that joint, sometimes fever, and almost always kidney stone complaints. It is characterized by higher blood levels of uric acid, one of the body's principle waste products. In a word, gout occurs when "the garbage isn't taken out on a regular basis."

A Peasant Medicine that Works Wonders

In 1979 I accompanied a number of other American scientists to the Soviet Union. There were about 40 or 50 of us and we were the special guests of the Soviet Academy of Sciences. This was back in the "good old days" of Communism, where in spite of its obvious corruption, a reasonable semblance of law and order existed. But since those times, the old USSR broke up into a number of smaller republic countries which went their own separate ways. Now in the infancy of Russian democracy, anarchy and crime appear to reign supreme, causing many older Russians to wish for less freedoms but a safer and saner society with the return of some kind of hard-line dictatorship.

Be that as it may, I had the opportunity during our historic month-long visit to that huge empire to meet with several old peasant-soldiers in the Ukraine who had somehow managed to survive the torturous gulags (prison camps) of the former Soviet leader, Joseph Stalin. These elderly man and their kind were once known as Cossacks and held special privileges in return for rendering military service to various Soviet leaders. Under the last of the old Russian czars they were often used to quell strikes and other disturbances.

Yani Dureyev, who was then 86 and as wrinkled as an old prune, with nary a tooth in his head, told me through an interpreter how his people always treated gout. They would make a type of vegetable

181

broth, using whatever was handy at the time. The soup would be strained and the clear broth saved, while the mushy vegetables would be fed to the pigs, ducks, geese, or chickens. Several large goblets (about 10 or 12 fluid ounces per goblet) of the broth would be drunk throughout the day. He claimed that there was always a cessation of gouty pain.

Using the scant information supplied to me in my interview with Yani, I finally managed to construct a reasonable facsimile of his old Cossack recipe.

COSSACK VEGETABLE BROTH

3 quarts mineral or seltzer water (Yani said it improves the flavor)

1 head of cabbage, coarsely chopped

1 onion, coarsely chopped

5 long stalks celery (with leaves included), chopped

1 bunch parsley, finely chopped

4 medium carrots (with tops), coarsely chopped

1 whole turnip (with top), coarsely chopped

$1/2$ beet with beet greens, coarsely chopped

some beef bones

Put everything into a large metal pot or kettle and cook over medium heat for $1 1/2$ hours. The vegetables by then should be quite mushy or completely broken apart. Remove from the fire and cool for 30 minutes. Then strain and refrigerate. Drink one cup every 4 hours or whenever gouty pains become severe.

Yani claimed that this remedy never failed to alleviate even the worst cases of gout.

Not Everything Russian Can Be Relied Upon

Not too long ago I read an article entitled "Soviet Sports Nutrition Secrets" in the November 1995 *National Foods Merchandiser* (p. 41) Nutrition Science News section (p. 9). A Russian biochemist by the name of Nikolai I. Volkov, Ph.D., was interviewed by Robert Hackman, Ph.D., an associate professor of nutrition at the University of Oregon in Eugene.

One of the subjects of discussion was natural things that would benefit athletes and trainers. Hackman asked Volkov if he had ever used any herbs during the 31 years he and his colleagues worked in Soviet sports nutrition research.

His Russian guest responded by saying the "we [had] developed . . . an herbal concentrate called *moomiyo*." He went on to describe how "moomiyo originates from junipers in the Himalayan mountains in central Asia." And that "decomposed juniper berries ° seep down into the rocks [and] after another 40 to 60 years the thick black paste is extruded from the rocks by geothermal pressure." After this, "gatherers scrape the paste from the rocks, refine it slightly to clean out the impurities, and that is moomiyo. Various grades of moomiyo exist."

The obvious reason (as I later learned) why Hackman had his Russian friend *deliberately* focus on the moomiyo aspects is because of attempts by at least one American company to market it here in the States. There is nothing wrong with this except that portions of Dr. Volkov's statements about this substance are simply *not* true.

Our group visited the former Soviet republics of Uzbek and Tadzhik during our visit there. In the city of Samarkand I met with several doctors, a geologist, and a biochemist. They were eager to tell me about *mumue,* the same stuff that Volkov mentioned to Hackman under the phonetic spelling of moomiyo. They even showed me some of it and made me a small present of several rocks of this hardened black, gooey stuff intact.

B-U-T, dear reader, the moomiyo that Volkov and Hackman would lead us to believe is made from decayed juniper berries over many decades is, in reality, *bat guano!* That's right, bat *excrement* from dark, dank caves high in the Himalayas. But, Volkov was correct in citing the methods of extraction.

In the Soviet Union in those times it was highly prized as a *medicinal* tonic for respiratory problems, autoimmune disorders, and joint inflammation. What all this should tell us is "don't believe everything you read," especially if it's marketing propaganda disguised as fact by clever hucksters in the gigantic health food industry.

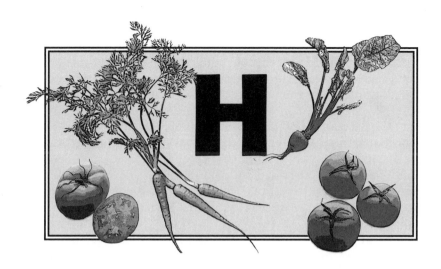

HEADACHE

Herbal Tea Secrets from the Tenth Annual Conference of the International Herb Association

DESCRIPTION

Heat is the principal *secret* here to making any of a number of herbal teas work for you in getting rid of a serious headache. *Warm* tea taken internally, *hot* herbal packs judiciously placed over the forehead and on the nape of the neck, and *hot* hand and foot baths all afford great relief from the pounding sensation of an awful headache.

Heat works because it seems to expand blood vessels, which constrict during a headache. Once better circulation is promoted this way, then the buildup of stress in the head eases and soon ebbs away.

Warm Teas for Relief

During July 27–30, 1995, the International Herb Association (IHA) held its tenth annual conference at the Palmer House Hilton in Chicago. There were more than 300 delegates present, comprising representatives of the herb industry, herb enthusiasts, and some scientists such as myself who have made it our lifetime profession of studying the wonderful effects of medicinal plants upon the human anatomy.

The event kicked off with bus tours to regional industry-related destinations such as the Morton Arboretum, the city's lovely Botanical Gardens, and many local herb businesses.

The keynote speaker was Mark Plotkin, Ph.D., who formally opened the first session with a spirited discussion on rain-forest conservation and the search for new medicines from the jungle. Plotkin is the author of *Tales of a Shaman's Apprentice* (New York: Penguin Books, 1993) and has conducted nearly all of his careful research with a number of different traditional folk healers throughout the world. A couple of days later, Varro Tyler, Ph.D., formerly the dean of the Schools of Pharmacy, Nursing, and Health Sciences at Purdue University in Indiana and author of several books on home remedies, delivered a rousingly good speech in the Otto Richter Memorial Lecture on the topic "Herbs and Healthcare: A Vision for the Twenty-First Century."

In conversation with each man, I obtained some interesting herbal "secrets" from them that jungle shamans and Indiana folk healers have utilized for a long time in getting rid of headaches. The following data are synthesized from both interviews.

Mix equal parts (one cup each) of water and apple cider vinegar in a pot and bring to a rolling boil. Then add $1^1/_2$ teaspoons of sage and $^3/_4$ teaspoon rosemary, stir, cover, and set aside to steep for 15 minutes. Strain and slowly *sip* one *very warm* cup of tea. Also, reheat some of tea until rather hot. Then soak a clean washcloth in it, gently wring out the excess liquid, and apply it across the forehead; do the same with another washcloth, then refold it and place under the nape of the neck. Cover the cloth over the forehead with a dry hand towel to retain the heat as long as possible; do the same with the folded washcloth under the neck. Change both when they become cool. Repeat treatment whenever headache recurs.

A medicine man from a remote Stone Age tribe still existing deep within the Amazon jungle made a tea of spider webs to relieve headaches in his patients. Plotkin claimed that as bizarre as it might sound, it *really* worked. The equivalent of one tablespoon of sticky cobwebs was stirred with a stick into what I judged to have been about 8 ounces of hot water and then slowly sipped. Plotkin reasoned that spider web must contain a substance that is good for the body's circulatory system and helps relieve headaches.

The Rest of the Convention

I mentioned to several of the delegates there, who were familiar with my work, that my own travels around the globe had turned up the use of *hot* peppermint tea, taken internally and used as baths in enamel pans in which to soak the hands and feet for effective headache removal.

Besides the conference's trade show and marketplace, organizers also had a trio of educational seminars running concurrently throughout the weekend. The first one dealt with the business of herbs and gave some savvy tips for their marketing. A second looked into the commercial production of medicinals and botanicals, offering small-scale herbal processors and manufacturers the most up-to-date information on procedures and techniques; this I found to be the most interesting of all. The third examined methods and means related to production and processing, from hydroponics to pest control, increasing herb yield and profits in greenhouse operations. I found this to be the most boring of all and walked out after 15 torturous minutes of endless babbling that seemed to go nowhere.

HEARTBURN

Fruit Juices and Herb Teas to Soothe
Burning Sensations

DESCRIPTION

The most common symptom for this disorder is a burning sensation in the middle of the chest. Other distinguishing features include pain and difficulty in swallowing, mild abdominal pain, and a slight regurgitation of stomach contents into the mouth, especially when the sufferer is reclining or bending forward.

Fruit Juices Help Cool the Fire

Heartburn can be due to several unrelated factors:

- narrowing of the esophagus (the passageway from the mouth to the stomach)
- gallbladder disorders
- gastroesophogeal reflux
- hiatal hernia
- peptic ulcer
- cirrhosis of the liver

Three of the best fruit juices I know of to help relieve the discomforts of these disorders are papaya, mango, and pear. One cup of any of these with a meal does wonders in preventing heartburn.

In the event, though, that a person suffering from heartburn has blood sugar problems and can't drink these juices because of their natural sugar contents, then several herb teas are recommended: chamomile, peppermint, or yarrow. Steep 2 tablespoons of any of them in 1 pint boiling water for 20 minutes, strain, then drink *lukewarm* with meals.

HEART DISEASE

Elixirs for Preventing Diseases of the Heart and Liver

DESCRIPTION

What is commonly called heart disease is also known in medical circles as valvular heart disease. The condition is characterized by damage to or a defect in one of the four heart valves: the mitral, aortic, tricuspid, and pulmonary.

Symptoms include shortness of breath and wheezing after limited physical exertion; swelling of the feet, ankles, hands, or abdomen; palpitations; mild chest pain; fatigue, dizziness or fainting; and occasional bacterial-induced fever.

Green Tea Affords Protection

A recent issue of *Food and Drink Daily* (Monday, March 20, 1995, p.4) carried an item of herbal interest from Reuter News Service of London, England. The dramatic headline read: "Green Tea May Protect Against Heart Disease." The article opened with a quote from Japanese research scientists claiming that green tea could help prevent both heart and liver disease.

A study of some 1,300 Japanese men over the age of 40 showed that the more green tea they drank, the more likely they were to have "healthy" levels of blood fats and other substances that can point to heart and liver disease.

Dr. K. Imai of the Saitama Cancer Research Center in Komuro was quoted to the effect that an "increased consumption of green tea was associated with decreased serum [blood] concentrations of total cholesterol." It seems that large intakes of tea each day help to increase the levels of "good" cholesterol (high-density lipoproteins or HDL).

Boil the water. Add the berries first. Cover with lid, reduce heat, and simmer for 5 minutes. Then remove the lid and add the green tea. Stir, replace lid, and set aside. After steeping for 10 minutes, uncover and add the hibiscus flowers. Stir again, cover and continue steeping for another 20 minutes. Strain and drink two cups daily with meals.

Iced Herbal Espresso for the Liver

This is a variation of an herbal tea remedy frequently recommended by Japanese kampo doctors to many patients concerned about the healthy state of their livers. Besides this, it makes a wonderful tonic for the skin. If prepared exactly as given below, a jet-black tea with an intensely bitter flavor will result. But if you dilute it, you'll get nearly the equivalent of iced brewed coffee. Some prefer it bitter, but others in Japan like to add some rice syrup, sugar, or honey to sweeten its flavor.

1 quart water

1¹/₂ tbsp. roasted chicory root

1¹/₂ tbsp. burdock root

1 cinnamon stick

2 tsp. green tea, loose and dried

Mix the first three ingredients together in a medium saucepan, cover with a lid, and simmer over low heat for 20 minutes. Uncover and add the cinnamon stick and green tea. Replace the lid and continue simmering for another 7 minutes. Set aside and steep for 20 minutes. Strain, add more water if necessary, and refrigerate. Drink one glass daily with a meal.

To help prevent heart and liver disease even further, it is a good idea to take one capsule each of dandelion and ginger roots and one capsule each of Kyolic EPA and Ginkgo Biloba Plus from nakunaga (see Product Appendix).

HEMORRHOIDS

Iced Tea Compress and Green Chlorophyll for Treating Piles

DESCRIPTION

Hemorrhoids, or piles, are nothing more than distended varicose veins in the anus. They itch, bleed, and can be painful during bowel movements.

How to Treat the Condition

Wash the anal area after every bowel movement. Use several layers of soft tissue for this. Fold them over and moisten under *warm* running water.

Then apply an iced tea compress for relief from itching and reduction of swelling and bleeding. This can be done in two different ways. Bunch together about 10 cotton balls to form one unit; dip this in iced green or black tea, gently squeeze out excess liquid, and then carefully insert between the buttocks. Change every five minutes. Or fold a clean, dry bath towel into a square and place on it an unfolded wet washcloth that has been dipped into some iced tea and then wrung out. Set both on a wooden or metal chair. Spread both buttock cheeks apart with the hands and slowly sit down on top of the towel and washcloth for about five minutes. Repeat this procedure twice again, but be careful not to get that part of the body too chilled.

Also, repeated applications of green chlorophyll liquid to the anal area are helpful. Mix 1 teaspoon of Pines wheat or barley grass juice concentrates with $1^1/_2$ cups of water. Dip 10 cotton balls bunched together or some folded soft tissue paper or a clean cotton cloth in the chlorophyll, squeeze out excess fluid, insert, and leave in place for 5 minutes. The chlorophyll can also be sprayed on or applied with a clean, thin brush.

HERPES ZOSTER

Oatmeal Water and Spinach Juice Work
Unbelievable Wonders

DESCRIPTION

Herpes zoster is the fancy name for the rather ordinary but potentially fatal disorder of shingles. It is caused by the identical virus that induces chicken pox, namely varicella zoster. When a young person gets over chicken pox the virus doesn't die but rather goes into long-term hibernation in the ganglion (sensory) nerve cells that extend from the brain to the spinal cord. Then, much later in advanced adult life the virus can be reactivated by a sudden mental or emotional trauma, too much stress, poor diet, or extremely cold or hot weather. It then migrates along the path of the nerve to the surface of the skin, where it causes a rash of painful blisters.

The outlook for recovery is good unless the virus has reached the brain. The treatments offered here are more for the relief of the blisters than for the actual cure of the problem.

Grain and Vegetable Treatments

Prepare some quick-cooking oats according to the instructions given on the label. But add *triple* the amount of water called for. Cover and set aside for seven minutes. Then strain the water and refrigerate, but discard the cooked cereal. Wash the herpes sores several times each day with some of the *cold* oatmeal water.

Martha Ames, a housewife from Worcester, Massachusetts, wrote me some time ago about how she used spinach juice for healing her elderly mother's herpes lesions. She made some spinach juice in her Vita-Mix whole food machine by blending together four leaves, $1/2$ cup water, and $1/2$ cup ice cubes for two minutes. The liquid in canned spinach may also be used, but doesn't work quite as well, she noted.

The best method of application she found after some experimentation was to paint on some of the juice with an artist's camel-hair brush that had never been used. "This, by far, is the easiest and most efficient way," she wrote. Fresh spinach juice was applied every four to six hours for a week or ten days.

She stated that it was "definitely very time-consuming," but that the pain diminished and healing became evident within a matter of days.

HIATAL HERNIA

(see Heartburn)

HIGH BLOOD PRESSURE

Hot Vegetable Tonic for Normalizing Blood Pressure

DESCRIPTION

Garlic has been widely utilized by many folk healers the world over for the treatment of hypertension. Clinical studies done with garlic extract have validated its use for this problem; in many cases a 65 to 83 percent improvement rate has been noticed.

Certain vegetables such as celery and green onion are high in the mineral potassium. A group of doctors and registered dietitians from the Second Medical School at the University of Naples in Naples, Italy, investigated the role of this important nutrient in the treatment of high blood pressure. And what conclusions did they finally reach? According to the November 15, 1991 issue of the *Annals of Internal Medicine* (115:753–59), "Increasing the dietary potassium intake from natural foods is a feasible and effective measure to reduce antihypertensive drug treatment."

Hot Drink Reduces Medication Needs

Those who have suffered from high blood pressure and regularly consumed this hot vegetable drink several times a week (three to four), reported wonderful improvements in their conditions, with a lot fewer prescription drugs.

HOT MIXED VEGETABLE TONIC

1 large tomato, quartered

1/4 cup celery

1/2 clove garlic

1 tbsp. liquid Kyolic Garlic (see Product Appendix)

1/2 green onion

1/4 cup carrots

1/4 cup hot water

Place all the ingredients in the Vita-Mix Total Nutrition Center container (or equivalent food machine) in the order listed. Secure completely the two-part lid by locking it under the tabs. Then move the black speed control lever to HIGH. Lift the black lever to the ON position and permit the machine to run for $2^1/_2$ minutes or until the contents are smoothly mixed. Makes 1 cup. Slowly drink while still warm.

To improve the flavor, add $^1/_2$ teaspoon granulated kelp (a seaweed) and an equivalent amount of Mrs. Dash (a commercial seasoning preparation); both are available from the spice section of most local supermarkets.

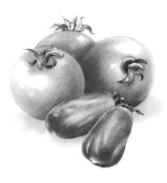

HOT FLASHES

Cooling Herbal Beverages from the Orient for Flushes

DESCRIPTION

Hot flashes are a common experience for about 85 percent of all women during their menopausal years. Hot flashes usually begin deep within the chest as an intense heat and soon radiate upward and outward through the shoulders, neck, and head. Not long after follows some degree of sweating.

At night a woman may be inclined to throw off her blankets, soak the sheets with sweat, then feel cold a few minutes later and require additional blankets. Hot flashes are a measurable phenomena. Skin surface temperature increases during a hot flash. A woman is very conscious of this and imagines that everyone can see her flushed skin. Such episodes end in a few moments and can recur within minutes or hours, depending on a variety of circumstances. Quite often there follows a short period of faintness or physical fatigue.

Cooling Down the Body

A number of American and European women I know who have found no immediate relief for this problem from Western medicine have elected to confer with Oriental herb doctors. They've told me that the best things that have helped them to cool down their flushed bodies are certain herbal teas, among them being Korean ginseng root, dong quai (tang kuei), fo-ti-teng (an herbal combination), and black cohosh root.

Through a lengthy process of trial and error many of the women discovered on their own that these herbs didn't work very well in pill, tablet, or capsule form. Some of them obtained a measure of relief using tinctures or fluid extracts of them. But their overall consensus was that the teas worked better for them than any other forms of these herbs did.

195

Preparing the Teas

1 1/2 pints water

1 1/2 tbsp. any recommended herbs (ginseng, dong quai, fo-ti-teng, or black cohosh)

Boil the water. Add only *one* of any of the previously cited herbs. Cover the pot with a lid, lower the heat, and simmer for approximately 7 minutes. Set aside and steep for 20 minutes. Strain and refrigerate. Drink one cup twice daily between meals.

Estrogen Substitutes

In her excellent book, *Women's Bodies, Women's Wisdom* (New York: Bantam Books, 1994; p. 446), Dr. Christiane Northrup wrote: "For women who are suffering from a combination of depression, sleep deprivation, and hot flashes, estrogen replacement can be very helpful, and I prescribe it regularly . . . ." She noted, however, that "it usually takes two to four weeks before estrogen therapy reduces hot flashes, though it may happen as soon as two or three days."

Two herbs I have routinely recommended over the years for hundreds of women going through menopause have been alfalfa and red clover. Both plants have an assortment of estrogenlike compounds that help to reduce hot flashes considerably. The standard for taking these herbs is a tea.

Estrogen Therapy in a Cup

4 cups water

1 1/4 tbsp. alfalfa herb

1 tbsp. red clover blossoms

1/4 tsp. pure vanilla flavor

1/4 tsp. honey to sweeten

Bring the water to a rolling boil. Add both herbs and stir. Cover with a lid, set aside, and steep 10 minutes. Uncover and add the vanilla. Replace lid and steep another 15 minutes. Strain, reheat, and add honey (optional).

Drink one cup of *warm* tea three times daily on an empty stomach. Continue this procedure of treatment for a month or longer, if necessary.

Supplement with Vitamin E

Dr. Northrup regularly prescribes Vitamin E in the form of alpha-tocopherol 400 I.U. two times daily for her patients who are being treated for hot flashes. But because nearly all the current forms of vitamin E on the market are either rancid or impure, I am hesitant to recommend any of them.

There is only one brand of vitamin E that I have been comfortable with for several decades now. My family and I have obtained much benefit from it, as have hundreds of others to whom I've recommended it. It is called Rex's Wheat Germ Oil, but has always been used primarily for domesticated livestock. However, just because it was made for animals doesn't mean it can't be used by humans, too. I suggest a woman troubled with hot flashes take one tablespoon of this oil each day *with food*.

Because this product is sold exclusively to veterinarians and livestock breeders, it isn't readily available to the general public. Therefore, as a public service our research center started offering it to the public *at cost* a while back. If you wish to order some Rex's Wheat Germ Oil for yourself, send $65 to the following address and allow up to two weeks' delivery time:

Anthropological Research Center
P.O. Box 11471
Salt Lake City, UT 84147

Please remember that this *isn't* a solicitation for your business. It is provided only as a service to interested readers who may not be able to obtain it otherwise on their own.

HUMAN PAPILLOMA

Grape Juice Strengthens the Immune System to Fight HP Virus

DESCRIPTION

In her book (previously cited under HOT FLASHES) Christiane Northrup declared that human papilloma virus (abbreviated HPV) is quite common, can produce venereal warts, and is frequently associated with abnormal Pap smears, or cervical dysplasia. She estimated that better than 50 percent of adult women and about 40 percent of children show some signs of HPV infection. The vast majority of women who have been exposed to HPV, she noted, don't develop any warts or cervical dysplasia, however.

Recently scientists have noted that some strains of HPV are more aggressive than others. And weak immune systems can definitely increase women's risks of acquiring this infection. When they do, painless warty growths *(condylomata acuminata)* on the outside of the vulva can be seen and felt. They can vary in appearance, from plaquelike growths to pointy, spiky lesions. HPV infection may also be associated with chronic vulvar pain, chronic vaginitis, and chronic inflammation of the cervix.

More women today have HPV because of liberal attitudes toward sex and the lifestyles that go with them. Condoms won't prevent the transmission of HPV, because the largest reservoir of the virus in the male is in the scrotum, and transmission is by physical contact. Even if a woman is monogamous, she can be exposed to warts depending upon the number of sexual partners that her own partner has had. Other factors believed to contribute to an HPV infection include weak immunity, poor nutritional habits, alcohol and drug abuse, cigarette smoking, and unhealthy emotions.

What Geneva W. Did for Herself

A friend of mine, a doctor I've know for years who regularly treats women infected with HPV introduced me to one of his patients a while back. Her name was Geneva W., age 43, white female, divorced, and working as a computer programmer for a large industrial plant in a major metropolitan area in the Midwest. The reason he thought I would be interested in talking with her by telephone is because of what she did to correct her HPV infection after all his own drug therapies had failed.

In our conversation sometime later, Geneva related to me that the various treatments my medical colleague had tried on her failed to stop HPV warts. "He couldn't laser the damn things off," she said. "Nor did a topical application of the antiviral medication Condylox (Podofilox) help very much either. And the TCA (trichloroacetic acid) just burned away the visible ones . . . it took my skin two weeks to heal again. I don't think I want to go through that hell again. Next he tried freezing them off with a cryocautery device, but it made them disappear for only about two and a half weeks, after which they came back with more of a vengeance. Finally, as a last resort, your doctor friend put me under anesthesia in a hospital operating room and tried burning the warts off with a heated electrical device; but this electrocautery didn't get rid of everything.

"Imagine how I felt at the end of all this," she continued. "I felt like a damned guinea pig and told him I was finished being used as some sort of experimental animal. I left and decided to take matters into my own hands after that."

She got hold of a book called *The Grape Cure,* written by a person many years ago who had actually been cured of malignant cancer by drinking nothing but dark grape juice. She said, "I figured, hey, I may not have cancer, but maybe this stuff might work just as well for me. So I bought a couple of bottles of Concord grape juice and started drinking two glasses of the stuff every day." In addition, Geneva also injected some of the grape juice into her vagina. "I couldn't see why douching with the juice would hurt anything," she stated with a laugh.

Nothing really happened for the first week or ten days. But "towards the end of the second week I began noticing a reduction in the warts on my cervix, vagina, and vulva," she observed. "I thought, wow, this stuff is great 'cause it seems to be working to *keep them from coming back again.*" This good progress intensified in the next several weeks. And within two months, Geneva W. reported back to my doctor friend, who was astonished to find her totally free of HPV-induced warts.

"That's my story he wanted you to hear," she concluded. "You may share this with others in your book, but I'd ask that you use only my first name and not mention where I work or live."

HYPERTENSION

(see High Blood Pressure)

HYPOGLYCEMIA

(see Mood Swings)

HYPOTHERMIA

Tomato Zinger for Raising Internal Body Temperature

DESCRIPTION

Hypothermia occurs whenever a person's internal body temperature drops below normal. Mild hypothermia is when body temperature ranges between 94°F. and 97°F., whereas more severe hypothermia is anything below 94°F. The lower the body temperature, the worse are the symptoms.

Symptoms of hypothermia include shivering, numbness, bluish or grayish skin tinge, slurred speech, confusion, stumbling, drowsiness, decreased pulse and breathing rates, dilated pupils, and loss of consciousness.

The elderly are the most vulnerable, since the ability to regulate body temperature diminishes with age.

Mexican Weather Forecast: Chili Today, Hot Tamale

Severe hypothermia can be life-threatening and requires emergency medical treatment! Mild cases, though, can be self-treated. If any wet clothing is on the individual it should be promptly removed and the person covered with dry clothing, quilts, or a down-filled sleeping bag. A stocking cap of some kind and gloves should also cover the head and hands. The person should lie down and rest.

The following hot vegetable drink, courtesy of the Vita-Mix test kitchen laboratory and slightly revised by me, is ideal for helping to restore body temperature back to normal. It is preferable to use a Vita-Mix Total Nutrition Center when making this and all juices or tonics mentioned in this book.

TOMATO ZINGER FOR REWARMING THE BODY

> *2 large tomatoes, quartered*
>
> *1 cup boiling water*
>
> *1 beef bouillon cube*
>
> *$^1/_2$ cup carrots*
>
> *$^1/_2$ cup celery, with leaves*

1/4 cup sweet red bell pepper

1/4 tsp. paprika

pinch of cayenne pepper

1 tsp. dried basil

Place all the ingredients in the Vita-Mix unit in the order given. Secure the complete two-part lid by locking under the tabs. Move the black speed control lever to HIGH. Lift the black lever to the ON position and allow the machine to run for $2^1/_2$ minutes, until smooth. Makes 2 cups.

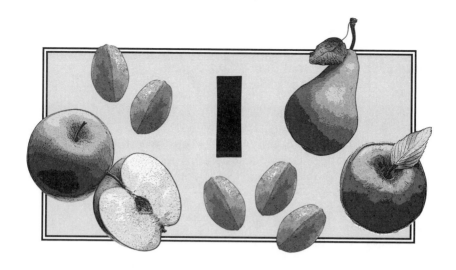

IMPOTENCY

(see Infertility)

INDIGESTION

Warm Herbal Teas Settle Upset Stomachs

DESCRIPTION

Indigestion can be caused by any number of factors. The first of these always seems to be eating in a hurry. Meals should be consumed in a leisurely manner and every mouthful thoroughly chewed. Second, one should never consume food while the mind is under stress or the emotions wrought up. Third, fluids should be consumed separately from meals, because they tend to dilute the saliva and hydrochloric acid produced by the body that are necessary for normal digestion. Also, unwise combinations of food can produce gastrointestinal discomforts; proteins and carbohydrates should always be consumed in separate meals. Finally, a person should never overeat, but should consume only that which satisfies, and the person should be able to leave the table still a little bit hungry.

Trolling for a Sandwich and a Cup of Tea

One in six Utahans has a fishing license, which equals about 300,000 people who fish and a whole lot of fishing stories. Some of the best of these stories can be heard at Chuck 'n' Fred's Cafe & Deli, a local diner owned by two fishing nuts. Chuck and Fred are so smitten with their sport that there is nary a square inch of their cafe, located at 2280 South West Temple in South Salt Lake, that doesn't celebrate the rod and reel in some way.

I was drawn to this local favorite eatery by a surgeon friend of mine with whom I occasionally golf. He is an avid fisherman himself and likes to frequent this place quite often.

We went there one Thursday afternoon, following a few rounds at the Jeremy Ranch Golf Course. I was intrigued with what greeted my eyes. For starters, there was a fishing boat mounted on the roof, emblazoned with the words "Try Us. You'll Get Hooked." Once inside, I found a weekly updated fishing report mounted on the wall space usually reserved for the daily specials. Chuck and Fred must have searched high and low for the trout-species-of-the-world wallpaper that serves as architrave for the front dining room. A stack of Polaroids was nestled in a rack alongside each menu, featuring a variety of strangers displaying various sizes of dead fish for the camera.

But hold on—there's more to relate. The back room, which seemed to be the hangout for Chuck 'n' Fred's regulars, was strewn with fishing caps of all kinds. And, as both owners told us, these are *reel* fishing caps, which carried the logos of local industries, not the kind made for holding expensive hand-tied flies. I was introduced to Chuck by my friend. As we shook hands, Chuck looked down at me and then up again, and said rather dryly, "Your fly's open." I looked down at my pants' zipper, but found it up all the way. He chuckled and replied, "That's my *catch* for the day, you falling for my joke and all."

As we seated ourselves at a booth and were handed menus by a gum-chewing waitress, I noticed a wooden sign hanging on the wall in the shape of a fish, with letters paint on it reading, "Try our fish just for the *hal-i-but* [helluv-it if you say it real fast]."

My doctor buddy had the "meatloaf surprise" with canned corn and instant whipped potatoes. "Why is it called 'surprise'?" I asked rather naively. "Because you gotta guess what we put into it," our waitress drawled as she made a loud pop with her bubble gum. I chose one of their quarter-pounders topped with mushrooms, bacon, hickory sauce, and cheese.

Halfway through our meal, my friend suddenly stopped and laid his fork aside, while at the same time putting his hand over his stomach. "Crap!" he snorted in disgust, "My gut is giving me problems again. I should know better than to have anything so greasy as this meatloaf." He drank a little ice water in between his moaning and groaning, but that seemed only to make matters worse.

I asked our waitress if they had any packaged herbal teas on hand. Much to my delight, she said they did and mentioned a choice between chamomile or peppermint. I selected the latter and had her bring *four* foil envelopes of teabags instead of the customary one or two. After she left us the tea and enough hot water, I put the bags into the large ceramic coffee cup and poured the water over them.

In about six minutes there was enough tea for the surgeon to drink. He carefully sipped the peppermint, remarking how delicious it tasted. Within 10 minutes he proclaimed with total satisfaction, "I feel 100 percent better. Thanks for the advice, John, and the great tea."

As we paid our meal checks at the cash register, Fred, the other owner, came out of the kitchen and said: "Remember, old fishermen never die, they just *smell* that way!" And with that we left.

INFERTILITY (MALE/FEMALE)

Removing the Emotional Pain and Raising Pregnancy Expectations

DESCRIPTION

For many young couples just getting married and hoping to start a family soon, the "All American Dream" could be handily summed up with this little ditty:

First comes love, then comes marriage,
Then comes Junior in a baby carriage!

But for about two in every dozen couples, those expectations can be quickly dashed when they learn that one or both may be infertile. After that there may be this:

Next comes sadness, then the fear,
And sorrows drowned in a keg of beer.

Couples I've known who, for whatever reasons, can't have kids are touched by a special kind of pain that can foul every aspect of their lives—how they feel about themselves, who they are, their bedroom relationship, even their marriage and their jobs.

One psychologist who specializes in marriage counseling, has told me that infertile couples have no sense of balance in their lives. He describes their experience as an emotional roller-coaster, up one week with hope and down the next with grief.

Natural Solutions that May Help

It would be nice if everything we attempted in life came with some sort of money-back guarantee like a lot of the products we buy. Unfortunately, that isn't always the case. But, at the very least, we can help increase our chances of things going right for a change, through prayer, persistence, and being willing to try something different.

Over the years I've been contacted by eleven different couples sharing a common problem: their infertility. I've recommended a juice-and-tea program for all of them that usually lasted about six months. Five of those couples realized single or multiple (twin) pregnancies, while the rest didn't. I'll be the first to admit that a 45 percent response rate doesn't sound very impressive at first glance. But considering that there is only a 20 percent success rate for most couples receiving conventional medical and surgical techniques for infertility, this other rate doesn't seem so bad after all.

The following recipes should be used regularly for half a year to guarantee young couples a higher success rate. It is important for *both* partners to follow the program. The two fruit/vegetable drinks can be alternated on separate days, while tea should be consumed seven times a week.

PREGNANCY PERFECTION

$1/_2$ cup celery

$1/_3$ cup red radishes

$3/_4$ cup fresh pineapple

$1/_2$ cup pineapple juice, room temperature

$1/_2$ cup ice cubes

Place all ingredients in a Vita-Mix whole food machine or its equivalent. Secure the lid, turn the unit on, and blend for almost 2 minutes, until smooth. Makes nearly two cups.

BABY BEVERAGE

$1/_4$ cup cranberry juice

$1/_4$ cup organic apple juice

$1/_2$ cup red cabbage, lightly steamed

1 cup instant beet juice (1 tablespoon of Pines organic beet root juice concentrate mixed with 1 cup of spring water; see Product Appendix)

$1/_2$ cup ice cubes

Place everything in the Vita-Mix Total Nutrition Center container or equivalent machine and secure the two-part lid in place. Turn the machine on and run for $2^1/_2$ minutes. Set aside for 30 minutes until contents are about room temperature. Remix on high speed for 1 minute, then drink. Makes close to $1^1/_4$ cups.

FAMILY-MAKER TEA

1 quart spring water (do not use tap water)
1¹/₂ tbsp. Korean ginseng root
1¹/₂ tbsp. sarsaparilla root
1 tsp. pure vanilla flavoring

Boil the water. Then add both herb roots. Cover and simmer on low heat for 15 minutes. Set aside and steep for 25 minutes. Strain and add the vanilla flavoring. Drink 1 cup *lukewarm* between meals 7 days a week.

SPERM ACTIVATOR

Take one tablespoon of Rex's Wheat Germ Oil each day with a slice of dark rye or pumpernickel bread for six months. To get a quart of this very potent Vitamin E supplement, send $65 to: Anthropological Research Center, POB 11471, Salt Lake City, UT 84147. An alternative is to take 400 IU of Vitamin E for two months, 600 IU for the next two, and 800 IU for the final two months.

INFLUENZA

(see Common Cold)

INGUINAL HERNIA

Herbal Teas that Help to Mend Abdominal Muscle Weaknesses

DESCRIPTION

A hernia or rupture appears in the body torso as a protrusion of soft tissue, such as a portion of the intestine through a weak spot in an abdominal muscle. The most frequent kind, an inguinal hernia, happens where the solar plexus meets the thigh in the groin region. Men are more apt to have this kind of rupture than women due to a residual weakness along the pathway (inguinal canal) where the testicles descended into the scrotum prior to birth. But any weakness in the abdominal wall can lead to this problem.

What My Father Has Done for Family Hernias

In self-help health books such as this one remedies mentioned are intended to either alleviate discomforts or to correct a problem wherever possible. Sometimes, though, medical expertise may also be warranted. If a hernia cannot be pushed back in and starts producing nausea, vomiting, loss of appetite, and abdominal pain, it generally requires immediate surgery. A strangulated hernia is terribly painful and needs prompt medical attention or the condition may prove fatal before long.

However, if a hernia is reducible or can be pushed back into the abdominal cavity and no serious symptoms prevail, then it *isn't* an immediate health threat and can either be self-treated or surgically repaired in the hospital at one's leisure.

Many years ago my father, Jacob, and my younger brother (by a year), Joseph Heinerman, were traveling from Salt Lake City down to south-central Utah where we then lived on a farm. Near what is called the Point-of-the-Mountain (where the Utah State Prison is located), my brother suddenly started feeling excruciating pain in the lower part of his abdomen. It hurt so badly that he started crying. My father pulled over the side of the freeway and stopped the vehicle. He got out and went around to the passenger's side and opened the door.

By then my brother was about ready to pass out. His skin color had turned an ashen gray. He pleaded with my father in a very weak voice, "Oh, Dad, please help me. I feel as if I'm dying." My father quickly unzipped my brother's trousers and reached his right hand down into the pants and beneath the underclothes. He quickly felt the bulge in the groin and slowly began working it back into the abdominal cavity with his fingers. Very soon the color came back into my brother's face again, much of the terrible pain ceased, and he felt tolerably better.

My father let my brother borrow one of his own old trusses that my dad has worn for many decades to hold in his own hernia. He then made several herbal teas that he had my brother take for the next six weeks. At the end of that time my brother's inguinal hernia had mended, and he required no further tea or the continued wearing of a truss belt.

My own experience with a hernia is recalled now for the reader's benefit. Around the time I was eight years old, our family was then residing in the small farming community of Salem in the southern end of Utah County. I was helping my father one summer remove a two-foot high wall of cemented cinder blocks encircling the perimeter of a rectangular concrete slab. I clearly remember swinging a heavy sledge hammer against this wall with my feet spread wide apart. After several days of doing this, I noticed a visible bulge develop in my right groin. I called it to my dad's attention, and he pronounced it as being an inguinal hernia.

He took me to Salt Lake City where I was measured and fitted for a truss that I had to wear for the next several months. I didn't like the idea of doing so, because it limited some of my physical activities and made it impossible for me to wear any shorts in the hot weather. During this time my father gave me several different kinds of herbal tea to drink. I wasn't too crazy about how they tasted but obediently complied with his wishes as the good son that I tried to be.

After approximately four months had passed, I was able to cease wearing that very much disliked rupture belt and didn't need to drink any more of those "nasty" teas either. My father took me to a naturopathic doctor who did a careful examination of my whole groin area and reported feeling or seeing *no* further evidence of any bulge. He gave me a clean bill of health, which pleased my father and me very much.

MUSCLE-REPAIRING TONICS

1¹/₂ pints boiling water
2 tbsp. slippery elm bark, coarsely cut and dried
OR
2 tbsp. mashmallow root, coarsely cut and dried
OR
2 tsp. fenugreek seed

Add the slippery elm bark to the boiling water, cover with a lid, and set aside to steep for 40 minutes. Strain and drink one cup twice daily on an empty stomach.

For the others, add either the root or seeds, cover with a lid, reduce heat, and simmer for 10 minutes. Then set aside and steep for 25 minutes. Then set aside and steep for 25 minutes. Strain and drink one cup twice daily between meals.

Continue this botanical therapy for up to six months, if necessary. It is also very helpful to wear some kind of a truss during this period. In the event that the inguinal hernia becomes more severe, be sure to seek the services of a qualified medical doctor *immediately.*

INSOMNIA

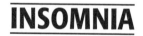

(see Nervousness)

ITCHING

Immediate Relief for Sensitive and Inflamed Skin

DESCRIPTION

General itching may or may not be accompanied by a rash. Unless it is disease-induced (melanoma or psoriasis) or parasitic-related (chiggers or ringworm), the following simple remedy will be of definite relief.

Willie Southall's "Quick Fix"

Several times each year I am a regular speaker for the National Health Federation conventions periodically held on different weekends at major cities around the country. A fellow speaker is a middle-aged African American from Los Angeles by the name of Willie Southall. He is a true believer in and heavy promoter of the herb hyssop.

When our speaking schedules weren't at the same times, I would occasionally drop in on some of his lectures, or he would attend a few of mine. At an NHF conference in Monroeville, Pennsylvania (near Pittsburgh), in the spring of 1995, I heard him telling his audience about the benefits of liquid hyssop for relieving itching skin. Willie explained how affected parts of the body could be sponge-bathed or sprayed with this herb for immediate relief. He called it his "quick fix for the itch."

He sells hyssop in different forms, including a liquid extract and what he calls a hysalgesic balm. They may be ordered by writing to Hyssop Enterprises, 7095 Hollywood Blvd., Suite 713, Hollywood, CA 90028.

ANTI-ITCH TEA

Or one can make a tea from coarsely cut, dried hyssop, which will work just as nicely. You may obtain it from most health food stores or herb shops or consult the Product Appendix for a mail order supplier.

1 pint boiling water

2 tsp. hyssop herb

Put the herb in the water, stir, cover with a lid, and set aside to steep for 35 minutes. Then strain and put into an unused plastic bottle with a spray applicator. Mist on the skin every three hours and watch the itching disappear.

Another remedy that is equally effective is tincture of witch hazel. This can be purchased from any drugstore or supermarket pharmacy section. Pour some of it into an empty spray bottle and put on the skin the same way. Both work well for the itching and inflammation that always accompanies sunburn. They can also be massaged into the scalp to relieve scalp itching.

JOCK ITCH

(see Itching)

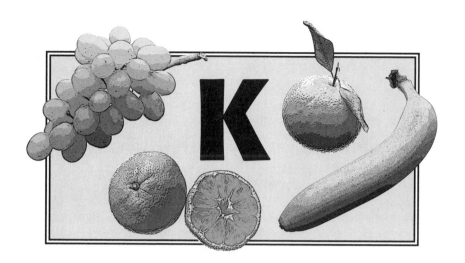

KIDNEY PROBLEMS

Rinsing Clean the Waste Filtration System of the Body

DESCRIPTION

The body's pair of kidneys are located on either side of the lower back. They regulate the fluid and electrolyte balance in the system and filter wastes out of the blood into the urine. Urine collects in the portion of the kidney known as the renal pelvis; from there is passes through a narrow conduit (the ureter) to the bladder.

Natural Rinses for the Kidney

The following natural substances help keep the kidneys in good working order.

BERRY-MELON CLEANSER

> *1 cup frozen raspberries, thawed out*
>
> *$^1/_2$ small watermelon, flesh scooped out of its rind and seeds removed*
>
> *ice cubes*

Place the raspberries in a Vita-Mix or equivalent food blender and process for one minute. Then add the watermelon and ice cubes and blend for another minute.

Yields about 4 glasses. Set aside somewhere in the kitchen until the chill has been taken off before drinking so as not to put the body in shock.

TEA RINSE

1 pint water

2 tbsp. kidney bean pods, coarsely chopped

OR

2 tbsp. cornsilk, dried

Add either herb, cover, and simmer for 3 minutes. Then set aside and steep for 25 minutes. Strain and drink 3 cups daily.

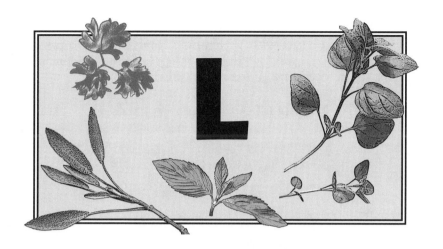

LABOR PAINS

End the Reign of Pain with Raspberry Leaf Tea

DESCRIPTION

Better educated women earning higher incomes usually report less labor pain. And older women report having less labor pains than younger women do. First-time moms tend to feel more pain than women who've had a few children. But the pain of childbirth, however difficult to bear, is considered rather benign since it is being experienced for a positive purpose (having a child).

Mother of 17 Has Pain-Free Deliveries

In my region of the country one of the common family surnames is Barlow—there are several thousand of them (besides Jessups and Johnsons). During the fall of 1995 and the spring of 1996, our family employed one of these Barlow men in the capacity of contractor to supervise a lot of construction work on our family ranch in the wilderness of southern Utah. This man came from a Mormon family of 63 children, fathered by one man through four different wives. His own mother had 17 children.

I was especially intrigued with one little detail mentioned in his narrative—his mother almost *never* experienced any of the labor pains so typically common for most other mothers. I got permission from his father to talk with the mother, one Martha Barlow. She explained to me how she used red raspberry tea to make all her deliveries "as easy as snapping your fingers," she said.

MARTHA'S TEA FOR PAINLESS LABOR

1 quart boiling water

4–5 tbsp. red raspberry leaves, dried

1 quart thermos bottle

Put the raspberry leaves into the boiling water. Stir, cover with a lid, and set aside to steep for 50 minutes. Strain and reheat. Then pour part of it into the thermos. Drink 1 cup every 3 hours in the last 5 to 9 days before expected delivery.

Martha insisted, however, that "it works only when the tea is taken somewhat *hot.*" It won't work if it's lukewarm or cool; *it must be almost hot* in order to be effective.

"I've had all my kids without nary a fuss," she boasted. "I've had some at home and others at the hospital. But I've never been without my raspberry leaf tea. It's the best thing for safe and hassle-free delivery. It truly is an expectant mom's best friend."

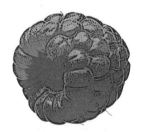

LACTATION (INADEQUATE)

Spicey Teas that Help the Milk to Flow

DESCRIPTION

One thing I've discovered in the last several years that has somewhat confounded me is the *inability* of many working women in America to properly breast-feed their own infants. One high-level female executive with a top sales organization told me once, "I just thought that breast-feeding was something any woman could do, not something that I had to actually *learn,* for heaven's sakes!" And yet, there are tens of millions of mothers in Third World countries all over the planet who just do it because it's second nature to them.

Herbal Spices to Promote Lactation

The following spices are good for breast milk production: anise, basil, caraway, dill, fennel, and parsley. They work best when drunk as *warm* teas.

> *1 pint water*
>
> *1¹/₂ tsp. basil or dill or parsley*
>
> **OR**
>
> *1¹/₂ tsp. anise, caraway, or fennel*

Boil the water. Then add the basil, dill, or parsley. Stir, cover with a lid, and set aside to steep for 35 minutes.

Or add the anise, caraway, or fennel. Cover and simmer on low heat for 5 minutes, then set aside to steep for another 25 minutes.

Strain and refrigerate. Reheat just enough for one-cup amounts. Drink *warm* tea with meals three times daily.

LEG ULCERS

Antibiotic Herbal Wash for Skin Breakdown

DESCRIPTION

Skin breakdown is a common and serious complication usually affecting bedridden senior citizens. Most common sites include elbows, hips, heels, outer ankles, and base of the spine. Over 95 percent of sores develop on the lower part of the body. They can be a result of anemia, diabetes, peripheral vascular disease, or dry skin, but mostly infections.

Appropriate Health Care the Natural Way

It is becoming painfully aware to many doctors that the era of "miracle antibiotics" is just about over. Today's new strains of super bacteria actually seem to thrive on such synthetic drugs. Only certain antibiotic herbs still seem to manifest a definite negative impact on these drug-resistant bacteria.

The two best herbs that work in such cases are garlic clove and goldenseal root. They make an efficient skin wash for leg ulcers in the elderly.

ANTIBIOTIC HERBAL WASH

1 $^1/_2$ pints water

1 tbsp. garlic clove, peeled and coarsely cut

$^1/_2$ tsp. powdered goldenseal root

Boil the water and add the garlic clove. Cover with a lid, reduce the heat, and simmer for 5 minutes. Set aside and steep for 10 minutes. Strain and return to pot. Add the goldenseal powder and stir in well. Cover with lid again and steep another 10 minutes.

Bathe the open leg sores 3 to 4 times each day using plenty of cotton balls and Q-tips, if necessary.

LIVER COMPLAINTS

Jump-Starting the Body's Most Important Organ with Dandelion, Carrot, and Tomato

DESCRIPTION

We're not talking any serious liver ailments such as cirrhosis, hepatitis, jaundice, or hepatoma (liver tumor). Instead, we're dealing with general liver malaise in this section. Below are some common signs of weak or malfunctioning livers:

abdominal pain and distension

dark circles around eyes

fatigue

fever

headache

lack of appetite

liver spots on backs of hands

pale complexion

puffy lower eyelids

unexplained weight loss

Dandelion—the Best Liver Herb I Know of

Of all the medicinal plants known to be useful for the liver, none has manifested such steady and consistent action as dandelion. All parts of the dandelion—flowers, leaves, and root—work wonders for restoring the body's most important organ to normal health again.

VICTORY JUICE FOR A HEALTHY LIVER

2 cups tomato juice, canned or bottled

1 cup dandelion greens, washed and cut

$^1/_2$ cup dandelion flowers, washed and cut

1 cup finely cut carrots

$^1/_2$ cup finely chopped celery, leaves included

$^1/_2$ cup finely cut green bell pepper, seeds included

2 spinach leaves, washed and cut

$^1/_2$ cup plain yogurt

1 tsp. extra-virgin olive oil

2 red radishes, washed and cut

1 tsp. granulated kelp (seaweed)

$^1/_2$ cup ice cubes

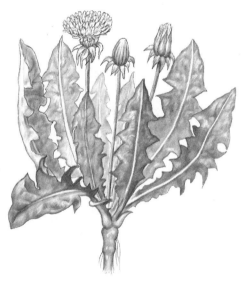

In a pot combine the tomato juice, dandelion greens and flowers, carrots, celery, bell pepper, and spinach. Cook over a medium heat setting until contents start to bubble a little. Then cover with a lid, turn the heat down to low, and simmer for 12 minutes. Set aside and let contents cool for 15 minutes.

Then transfer this mixture to a Vita-Mix container or equivalent food machine. Add the radishes before securing the two-part lid in place by locking it under both tabs. Move the black speed control lever to HIGH and lift the black lever to the ON position for 2 minutes. Set aside to cool some more in the container. Then return it to the machine and add the yogurt, oil, kelp, and ice cubes. Blend for another 1$^1/_2$ minutes. Makes a little over two glasses. Drink one glassful each day with a meal.

Dandelion may also be taken in capsule form. I advise taking two capsules of powdered dandelion root every day with a glass of water or vegetable juice. You'd be amazed how much this can help to rejuvenate an ailing liver. And you'd be even more astonished if you added two capsules of ground turmeric root with it. You can buy the turmeric in any supermarket spice section. But you'll need to hand fill the capsules yourself, since no herb company I know of sells turmeric in this form. You can get the gelatin capsules from most pharmacies or drugstores. I recommend putting the turmeric into capsules rather than taking it straight, because of its bad taste.

Dandelion root tea has always been an old reliable standby used by herbal folk healers the world over for treating many difficult liver disorders. You can buy the root either from any health food store or already packaged from an herb shop. Or go out and dig up some from your front lawn or back yard or vacant field or city lot. Just be sure that these areas haven't been sprayed with pesticides. Use a small digging trowel to get the roots out. Wash them off, slice diagonally with a sharp knife, spread out on an old, clean bedsheet, and allow to dry in a room of your house or apartment that receives frequent heat and is the warmest. Store in a glass fruit jar with screw-on lid and use when needed.

DANDELION LIVER TONIC

1 pint spring or distilled water

2 tbsp. dandelion root

1 cup mineral water

Boil the water. Add the roots, cover, and simmer on low heat for 10 minutes. Set aside to steep for 20 minutes. Strain, add the mineral water, and refrigerate. Drink one cup a day between meals.

Tomato Juice—Bugle "Wake-Up" Call for the Liver

Some years ago and old D.I. (drill instructor) for the United States Marine Corps (since retired) told me, with a malicious chuckle, how he used to get his "grunts" (new recruits) out of bed if they tried to oversleep. "I'd have one of the guys from the bugle corps come over and blow reveille directly into their ears. I guarantee you one thing, *no one* in my platoon ever dared to oversleep so long as I was around."

Well, I've come up with the juice equivalent for this to help arouse your sluggish liver.

LIVER WAKEUP CALL

1 cup tomato or V-8 juice, canned or bottled (low-sodium)

1 cup fish stock (optional) (made by cooking fish bones in one pint of water 30 minutes and then straining and refrigerating)

1/2 cup ripe tomato, quartered

1 tsp. Pines wheat grass juice concentrate (see Product Appendix)

1 tsp. liquid Kyolic Garlic from Wakunaga (see Product Appendix)

3 tbsp. plain yogurt

1/2 tsp. lemon juice

1/2 tsp. lime juice

pinch cayenne pepper

Combine everything in the order given in a Vita-Mix Total Nutrition Center or equivalent food machine. Process for 3 minutes or until smooth. Yields almost 3 cups.

Ale for an Ailing Liver

Common sense says that alcohol isn't good for cirrhosis of the liver or for fatty liver degeneration, yet for other common liver and gall bladder complaints a little—and the key here is *little*—bitter, brown and stout ale may be efficacious. Such ale has tremendous vitamin B value in it, not to mention a lot of enzymes, too. They work medicinal magic on an ailing liver, spleen, or gall bladder. For more information, please consult the next entry of MALNUTRITION.

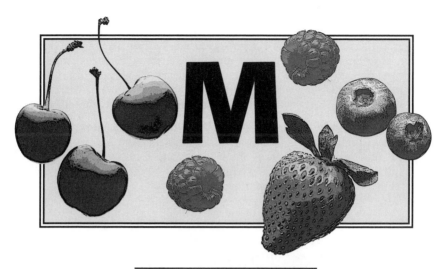

MALNUTRITION

Health Magic in Brewed Beverages

DESCRIPTION

Crafted brews got their real start in America in 1965 when business entrepreneur Fritz Maytag, using some venture capital funds, bought the Anchor Brewing Company of San Francisco and launched Anchor Steam Beer, a full-flavored, all-malt amber. Then in 1979, Charles Finkel began to import the *créme de la créme* of European beers: the full line of Samuel Smith's British ales and the Belgian Trappist ales. They became an instant hit with beer lovers from coast to coast.

But strange to say, those who switched to such brews and drank them in *moderation* (no more than one bottle every two days) made a surprising discovery: They began to feel better and have more energy. A few doctors who've studied this little known phenomenon attribute the health-giving properties of these crafted brews to their traditional ingredients (all of which are natural, by the way): malted barley, yeast, top-quality hops (a conelike flower that imparts bitterness and zest), and water.

The wide diversity of styles is usually determined by the different yeast strains, fermentation temperature, the degree to which the malt itself is being roasted, and the amount of hops intended to be used. The two basic types are:

ALES: Top-fermented—where the yeast rises to the top of the vat as the beer ferments, usually at moderate temperatures. Ales range from pale gold to dark amber and are generally more pronounced in flavor than lagers. Styles would include Porter and Stout, which can be higher in alcohol (up to 8 percent) than other ales.

LAGERS: Bottom-fermented—wherein the yeast settles to the bottom of the vat, at colder temperatures, and the brew is permitted to take a few weeks of very necessary vacation rest before being shipped out. Styles include these: Pilsner—light, gold; Bock—dark, malty (with a very unmistakable hop flavor); Double Bock—extra malty, darker, and higher in alcohol.

These ales and lagers can be obtained at most state-run liquor stores or at some delis and supermarkets. Or you can obtain them, believe it or not, by mail order: just call Ale-in-the-Mail at 1-800-573-6325. But remember, it's intended only for *medicinal* purposes and not for recreational drinking.

Istanbul Cab Driver Counteracts Malnutrition with Turkish Brew

Some years ago when I was in the foreign city of Istanbul on brief business, I hired a taxi for several hours to take me around to the different places I had to go. Fortunately for me my driver spoke some English, but I was not so lucky that he drove like a bat out of hell.

He drove at what I considered to be Mach II speed (something akin to what Air Force jet fighter pilots are used to), zipping through back alleys and preferring the blast of his loud horn to the more prudent option of applying brakes.

He gave his name as Ihtiyarlar Meclisi; I asked him to spell it out slowly for me as I wrote it down. But to this day, I still can't remember how to pronounce the darned thing correctly. So, I'm just going to refer to him by the nickname that he preferred to be called, *Yarla*.

Anyway, during our several hour-long rides together, we had a chance to visit a lot and conversed on all sorts of things. He showed me some old color photos of himself, apparently taken a few years before we met. It showed an emaciated figure with dark-brown skin stretched loosely hanging over his bony frame. At that time he suffered from obvious tissue wasting, loss of subcutaneous fat, and some dehydration due to critical deficiencies in both calories and protein. Because his family was poor, they could not afford to employ the services of a doctor to try and find out exactly what he may have suffered from.

His father, however, knew of a muhtar (headman) who was in charge of a village commune some distance on the outskirts of sprawling Istanbul. His father consulted this old man, who knew a thing or two about folk healing. The muhtar suggested that Yarla start drinking a beverage called *Kaza,* which is a locally made dark lager preferred by many Turks. It is relatively cheap and readily available; I bought a bottle and tried it myself. While admittedly rather bitter, it seemed to improve my digestive tract and gave me more energy. But more than one bottle of that stuff and I would have probably been seeing double due to the high alcohol content.

Well, as Yarla told it, his father started buying bottles of this stuff and had his son drink small amounts of one bottle each day with every meal. Yarla discovered that he could again start eating many of his favorite foods without constantly vomiting them up. He returned to a diet consisting of cooked barley, potatoes. grapes, olives, hazelnuts, mutton, and goat meat.

After following this liquid therapy for several months, he put on weight, improved his complexion, gained strength, and felt better than he had in some time, he declared in broken English.

An Ale for What Ails You

My crazy cab driver felt compelled to exert his virility by gunning his fiendish machine around the back alleys and side streets of Istanbul. It is true that we avoided main traffic congestion, but, oh, at what expense to my nerves and stomach! He dashed between a deluge of buses, lorries (trucks), motorbikes, horse-drawn carts, and other taxis without so much as blinking an eye. The sight of a poor pedestrian looming ahead of us motivated Yarla only like a shot of adrenaline, spurring him into quick action to accelerate and take aim.

Agile pedestrians deepened his macho insecurities. As we sped by he cursed the offending parties in native Turkish and made obscene gestures while leaning out of his window. I asked him what several of them meant, but the explanations offered were so crude that my publisher wouldn't let me include any of them in this book for fear of offending sensitive readers. These gestures, of course, required him to take both hands off the steering wheel. He used his left knee to steer while his right foot continued to press the accelerator through the floor. I was glad when my flight took off from Istanbul the next morning, putting considerable distance between me and my "cab ride from hell." However, I think I met up with one of Yarla's cousins when I landed at Kennedy International Airport in

New York City and hailed the first yellow cab, driven by a man from Turkey, of all places.

But the remedy I picked up from this guy in Istanbul was in direct contrast to the incredible stress I had to go through while riding around with him to my various appointments. I started drinking dark British ales myself whenever dining on red meat or eating heavy meals. I discovered how much easier my food digested as a result of this. And I began recommending to many older people, *one cup* of dark ale every day with their *afternoon* meals. Many of them who started doing this on the strength of my suggestion reported back later on how much better they felt overall and how better nourished they seemed to get from the food they regularly ate. From their personal and my own experiences with ales, I would have to say that these crafted brews exert a positive influence for good on the liver, gall bladder, and spleen, provided that they are taken in *moderate* amounts, say *one cup* per day.

Liquid Aloe Vera

Aloe vera is a plant of great historic importance renowned for its healing of inflamed tissue. Factors within the gel tend to inhibit the action of bradykinin, a peptide that produces pain in injuries such as burns. Aloe gel also inhibits the formation of thromboxane, a chemical detrimental to wound healing.

Aloe vera is available in liquid form and can be taken in small amounts (one-quarter cup every day) or mixed with a variety of fruit and vegetable juices in greater quantity (one-half cup). It is recommended in cases of malnutrition where nutritional rehabilitation is most desirable. Liquid aloe vera encourages enzyme activity within the gastrointestinal system, which helps to promote better digestion and, ultimately, better assimilation of the nutrients found in consumed food.

MENOPAUSAL SYMPTOMS

(also see Hot Flashes)

also:

MENORRHAGIA

MENSTRUAL PERIOD (ABSENCE OF)

(see Amenorrhea)

MENSTRUATION (HEAVY)

(see Menorrhagia)

MIGRAINES

(also see Nervousness and Stress)

MISCARRIAGE

MOOD SWINGS

MORNING SICKNESS

Irish Hospitals Prescribe World-Famous Local Brew for Wide Variety of Ailments

DESCRIPTION

Seldom have I classified so many different but interrelated health problems together in one section in any of the health books written by me in the past. But by a good stroke of luck, I was pointed in the direction of Dublin, Ireland, through my editor and good friend at Prentice Hall, Douglas Corcoran.

In one of our fairly regular phone chats together he told me on Sunday, November 12, 1995, from his home in New Jersey about his visit to the United Kingdom some time in 1972. "I had just graduated from college and was touring Europe with some friends. We were in the city of Dublin, where I happened to develop a bad case of bronchitis. So I went to King's Hospital to get some prescription medication for my problem. While sitting outside the pharmacy waiting for it to be filled, I noticed a nurse pushing a cart down the hallway to one of the hospital wards. There were about 20 to 30 glass mugs filled with a dark beer.

"I thought to myself, 'What one earth is going one here?' I asked this woman where she was taking all of this beer. She cheerfully replied, 'Oh, we give some of this to our patients every afternoon; they can't do without it. We think the Guinness Stout is pretty good medicine for them.' I was so intrigued by what I had just seen that after I got my medication my friends and I headed on over to the Guinness Brewery, where we got a royal tour of the facilities and some free pint glasses of their Extra Stout to sample. I must say that after drinking the stuff it seemed to be as nourishing to me as any home-cooked meal would be. There was almost a 'wholesome nutrition' to it, besides tasting smooth and robust. It was as if I had just consumed *a liquid meal of total nourishment!"*

Four Dublin Hospitals Contacted

This conversation inspired me to contact four of the five major hospitals in Dublin myself by telephone on Tuesday, November 14. The calls were placed between 2:00 and 3:00 P.M. Mountain Standard Time, which made it between 9 and 10 P.M. Dublin time. The four area hospitals were James Conley Memorial Hospital in Blancharstown (a suburb of Dublin), King's Hospital, Coombe Women's Hospital, and Holles Hospital (all located in Dublin proper).

I am grateful to Anne Flaherty, R.N., Lorraine Kyen, M.D. (Medical Registrar), Francois Gardiel, M.D. (Medical Registrar), Shawn Eliot, Ph.D., and several members of the senior medical staffs of two of these four hospitals (who didn't wish to be identified in this book) for their kind cooperation and assistance. They provided me with a lot of valuable information concerning the medical use of Guinness Extra Stout and similar Irish beers, which filled up several lined pages of extensive notes taken as I spoke with each of them.

A brief sideline of humor ought to be mentioned here in connection with this bit of research. When I spoke with Lorraine Kyen in the A & E (Accident and Emergency) section of James Conley Memorial Hospital, she paused to speak with some of her colleagues around her. I could hear faint laughter in the background and inquired as to its meaning. She replied with a chuckle, "Some of my fellow co-workers here in the casualty department, who can overhear what I'm telling you, think that our conversation is a lark and a bit strange."

I responded: "Tell them that you're talking to one of those crazy Yanks here in America. They'll understand since we're looked upon as being a little odd anyway by folks over there." She laughed good-naturedly, and our discussion of the medicinal benefits of Guinness Stout continued.

I was surprised to learn from Dr. Gardiel that the Guinness Brewery has had "a lengthy historical relationship" with Coombe Women's Hospital in terms of financial grants as well as by Guinness supplying the hospital with its dark brew for obvious medicinal purposes. By the way, this is the same company that has sponsored, for many years, the publication of the famous *Guinness Book of World Records.*

Medicinal Applications

Guinness Extra Stout is imported directly from the Dublin brewery and may be obtained in bottles at most state liquor stores, finer eating establishments with bars, or upscale private clubs. Or you may write or call the company's American agent for more information on how to obtain some of it:

Guinness Import Company
6 Landmark Square
Stamford, CT 06901
(203) 323-3311

The following information was condensed from my copious notes taken in my telephone interviews with the different doctors, nurses, and other health care professionals who work at the various hospitals contacted. I've also included some other things that may be of additional help as well.

Menopausal Symptoms. One-half cup of imported Guinness Extra Stout with breakfast. If this poses a problem, however, with your employment or driving due to the alcoholic content, then take the same amount with a meal in the evening when you come home and don't have to drive anymore.

Women entering menopause need to understand that it is *more* psychological stress rather than physical stress that brings on menopausal symptoms. Some anthropologists such as myself and Ann Wright have proven this in our own individual studies of certain Native American tribes of the American southwest. I've studied the Hopi and Zuñi tribes of Arizona and found little or no menopausal symptoms to speak of. Ann Wright looked for menopausal symptoms in reservation and city-dwelling Navajo women and made comparisons between the two groups. In an article she wrote for *Changing Perspectives on Menopause* (Austin: University of Texas Press, 1982), edited by Ann Voda, Myra Dinnerstein, and Cheryl R. O'Donnell, Dr. Wright mentioned that reservation Indian women had "very few symptoms." But those who were acculturated and living in the white man's world manifested just as many symptoms as other American women do.

I recommend that a woman drink catnip, chamomile, or peppermint teas or any of the wide range of herbal blends currently on the market to help lessen tension and anxiety in today's chaotic and fast-paced world.

Menorrhagia. Women who experience abnormal blood loss during heavy menstruation are at greater risk to suffer anemia. Tests conducted on Guinness Extra Stout and other Irish beers have shown them to be exceptionally high in iron content. One-half cup taken twice daily *with meals* or with several pieces of whole-grain bread will resupply a woman with much of the iron her body needs during this critical biological period.

A tea made from amaranth or pigweed, shepherd's purse, sorrel, or yarrow will help to stop excessive bleeding. Drink 2 cups a day during this period. Or take 2 capsules of goldenseal root or 10 drops of fluid extract of birthroot twice daily.

Migraines. At Coombe Women's Hospital Guinness Extra Stout has sometimes been recommended to those older men or women suffering migraine headaches that are due *primarily* to food- or drink-related allergies. In such instances, one-quarter to one-half cup of Guinness is taken by the patient every four hours. And, as awful as *warm* beer sounds (and tastes), as efficacious it is in helping to reduce bad headaches of this type. The brew can be warmed in a mug placed in a pan of boiling water over heat for about five or eight minutes. The beer should *not* be hot, only lukewarm.

A tea made from any of these herbs or spices will help alleviated a migraine rather nicely: balm, basil, cleavers, fennel, lavender, nettle, peppermint, primrose, rosemary, shepherd's purse, valerian, wormwood, and yerba maté. But the tea needs to be taken *warm* in order to be of any effect.

Miscarriage. About one in six pregnancies ends in miscarriage. And several clinical studies have demonstrated that in women who have repeated (three or more) miscarriages, there often is an interplay between emotions and the hormonal systems involved in pregnancy.

At Coombe Women's Hospital prospective moms are encouraged to take one-quarter cup of Guinness Extra Stout each day with a meal *after* the first trimester (three months) of pregnancy. I recommend that after the first quarter of fetal development that a mother-to-be drink one cup of chamomile tea daily and one cup of Kyo-Green from Wakunaga as well (see Product Appendix for more details on how to get this).

Mood Swings. Emotional highs and low are usually diet-related. They are common in many cases of hypoglycemia and yeast infection. Ordinarily the consumption of alcohol is detrimental in such cases. But not so at Holles Hospital in Dublin, where some doctors have prescribed *a little* Guinness Extra Stout for their patients suffering from low blood sugar. The key here is to take this in *small* amounts, *never* exceeding more than $1^1/_2$ cups for the entire day. They should be measured out in one-half-cups amounts morning, noon, and night and should *always* be taken *with food* and *never on an empty stomach.*

Also, the following juice recipe is very helpful in leveling out personal moods so that they don't swing from one extreme of ecstatic joy to the other end of manic depression or sudden anger.

Good-Mood Juice

3 ripe tomatoes, quartered

$^1/_4$ cucumber, washed, peeled, and quartered

1 large red radish, shredded on a metal grater

1 whole purple cabbage, leaves cut up

$^1/_2$ cup spring water

Place everything into a Vita-Mix Total Nutrition Center or equivalent food machine and secure the two-part lid by locking it under both tabs. Turn the machine on and run for 1 minute. Makes about $1^3/_4$ cups.

Morning Sickness. At King's Hospital in Dublin some OB/GYN (obstetrics and gynecology) doctors routinely prescribe some Guinness Extra Stout to those women who suffer from a great deal of nausea during the first part of their pregnancies. The women are advised to *slowly sip small amounts* (no more than one-quarter cup at a time) Guinness Extra Stout whenever nausea occurs. Because of the heavy enzyme activity in the dark stout, it usually helps settle the digestive system and eliminate any queasy feelings.

A *lukewarm* tea made from any of the following herbs and *slowly* drunk will help to settle an upset stomach: anise, caraway, chamomile, clove, ginger, red raspberry, sage, savory, or spearmint.

TEA PREPARATION

1 pint spring or distilled water

1$^1/_2$ tsp. of any of the aforementioned herbs

Boil the water. If the herbal material is seeds, bark, or root, then after adding it to the water cover with a lid and simmer on low heat for 5 minutes. Then set aside and steep for 25 minutes. Strain and drink one-half to one cup of *warm* tea, sweetened with honey or pure maple syrup, if necessary, to improve the flavor.

But if the botanical substance is of more delicate nature, such as flowers or leaves, then add the material, stir with a spoon, cover with a lid, and set aside to steep for 30 minutes. Strain and drink per previous instructions.

Stout Ales and Beers Good for the Elderly

I was astonished when most of my medical informants told me that a large number of their elderly patients prefer taking one-half to a full *bottle* of Guinness Extra Stout or something equivalent prior to retiring for the night. They claim it helps them to sleep a lot better.

Another thing that seems to help older people a lot after drinking a bottle of some stout ale or beer is the *increased* energy they claim to experience. Doctors whom I spoke with through a number of international telephone calls that cost me a mint verified this for me. Their observations have been that such elderly folks manifest more vigor and vitality than those few who are teetotalers for personal or religious reasons.

What Makes Guinness Stout Such a Health-Giving Drink?

I contacted some of the people at the Guinness Brewery in Dublin a few days later and at a more reasonable hour for them (10:00 A.M. over there) but at an awful time for me (3 A.M. in the "bloody" morning (as they say in Ireland). They gave me a brief history of their facilities. Arthur Guinness brewed his first stout in 1759. Sir Benjamin Lee Guinness, who became the first lord mayor of Dublin, developed a large export trade of porter and stout beers to America, England, and the rest of Europe.

The ingredients have been a closely guarded secret for several centuries. But I was reassured by the folks at Guinness that the original recipe has *not changed once* in all that time. With a bit of persistence, however, I managed to prevail long enough to draw out of them the following comments.

In all honesty, I must confess that one of the first things said was "You're a bit of a pushy Yank, aren't you?" The *three most important* ingredients critical to success of robust and mellow Guinness that is always smooth and satisfying are the *barley,* the *yeast,* and whatever kind of *mineral salts* are added to the water. The hop flowers and several other herbs are somewhat secondary, believe it or not.

What is known as two- or six-row malted barley is made by soaking whole barley seeds—including their husks—for several days under controlled conditions so that they sprout or germinate. During the soaking phase, the protein contained in the bran of this barley is converted into enzymes that change the starches to sugars. Then the barley is dried to prevent further sprouting. Theoretically, though, this process would work with any grain, but barley is well suited to malting because the bran layer is particularly rich in proteins that form many complex enzymes in the sprouting process. The conversion of starch to sugar creates the conditions necessary for fermentation by yeast, which produces alcohol.

Guinness differs from other breweries in the *number* of *different* barleys used to make their stouts. Roasted barley is added to increase the robustness. And chocolate malt (a specifically malted type of barley) is added for darker and thicker flavor. And only the brewmaster knows which kind and how much mineral salts to add to the water.

Barley happens to be one of the most nutritious cereal grains around. A soup or stew, with or without meat, made from barley provides a substantial one-dish meal. The variations on barley soup are endless; undoubtedly the most familiar are mushroom-barley and beef- or lamb-barley combinations. Mushroom-barley soup can be made with lamb, goat, beef, or chicken, or with just vegetable stock or water, and dried mushrooms, which give it a nice rich flavor. A very popular Polish barley soup called *krupnik* also contains dried mushrooms as well as potatoes and dill. A bowl of meatless barley soup can be enhanced by a dollop of plain yogurt.

Round out any barley soup or stew with lots of chopped vegetables. Those that seem to work the best here are leeks, onions, chives, carrots, parsnips, turnips, and cabbage. Scotch broth is a classic example of how such vegetables can be ingeniously combined with lamb to create quite a mouth-watering dish.

The following table gives the most important nutrients for one-half cup (3.5 oz.) cooked pearl barley.

Vitamin B-6	0.3 mg.
Copper	0.5 mg.
Folacin	19 mcg.
Iron	4 mg.
Magnesium	133 mg.
Manganese	1.9 mg.
Niacin	5 mg.
Phosphorous	264 mg.
Potassium	452 mg.
Riboflavin	0.3 mg.
Thiamin	0.6 mg.
Zinc	3 mg.

MULTIPLE SCLEROSIS

Oil and Water *Do* Mix in this Tonic Treatment

DESCRIPTION

Multiple sclerosis happens when the nerve casings, known as myelin sheaths, lose their protective outer fatty layer that insulates the nerves themselves and increases the speed of electrical transmissions. In multiple sclerosis (MS), patchy areas of these sheaths are destroyed (demyelinated) and replaced by scar tissue (called plaques)—a process know as sclerosis—at multiple sites throughout the central nervous system (hence the name of this disorder).

Some of the most common symptoms include extreme fatigue, spasticity in the arms and legs, muscle spasms, blurred and double vision and some eye pain, pins-and-needles sensation in the lower extremities, loss of physical coordination, vertigo, slurred speech, depression and mood swings, mental confusion, and partial facial or body paralysis.

A Tonic Different from What You May Expect

The following recipe (courtesy of the Vita-Mix Corporation) has been slightly revised by myself to include two plant oils essential for the restoration of myelin sheaths in MS recovery. After some kitchen experimentation with various recipes, I chose this one because it seems to be the best juice medium for both oils. It can be taken *warm* with a meal or by itself.

RECOVERY COCTAIL FOR MS

1 cup creamed corn

1 medium carrot, peeled

1 tbsp. liquid Kyolic Garlic (see Product Appendix)

2 green onions (chives)

1 cup milk, hot (preferably goat milk)

$1/4$ tsp. dry mustard

$1/4$ tsp. paprika

1 tsp. flaxseed oil

1 tsp. evening primrose oil

OR (if unavailable)

1 tsp. Rex's Wheat Germ Oil ($65 per quart from Anthropological Research Center, POB 11471, Salt Lake City, UT 84147)

1 chicken bouillon cube

white pepper, to taste

Place all ingredients in a Vita-Mix Total Nutrition Center or equivalent food machine container in the order given. Secure the lid and run the machine for up to 3 minutes until the contents are smooth. Makes slightly over 2 cups.

The following tea is also worth pursuing and delivers results that will greatly surprise you.

MIXED-SEED TEA

1 pint boiling water

1 tsp. raw sunflower seeds (dehulled)

1 tsp. fenugreek seed

Add both seeds to water. Cover with lid and simmer on low heat for 10 minutes. Set aside and steep for 20 minutes. Strain and drink one cup with a meal.

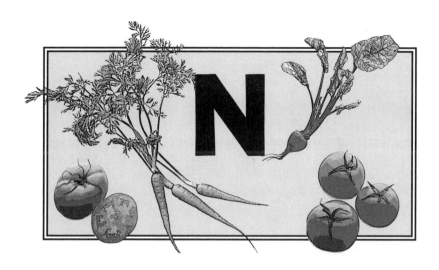

NERVOUSNESS

Anxious Councilwoman Calms Her Jittery Nerves with Some Peppermint Tea

DESCRIPTION

Every so often elections are held between political opponents that end with each side getting an identical number of votes. When this happens a recount is usually in order. But what if the recount turns up the same amount of votes for each?

This is precisely what happened between Diane Layton, age 43, an incumbent on the Clearfield (Utah) City Council and her opponent, David W. Monson, age 54. On November 7, 1995, 854 votes were cast for each candidate during statewide elections. A local CPA (certified public accountant) firm was ordered to re-count every ballot carefully in the event there might have been a miscount somewhere. They too came up with 854 votes apiece.

From here on the suspense heightened and things became even more interesting.

Tea Kept Me from Becoming a Basket Case

Utah state law then kicked into action. Statutes required that when such ties in voting occur a clear winner must be determined by lot. Incumbent Layton confessed to me that she was getting the jitters wondering whether or not she would be able to retain her seat on the city council.

"I was never so nervous in my life," she admitted. "I had butterflies in my stomach the whole time." To help settle her frayed nerves, her grandmother recommended that she drink some warm peppermint. "I found this to really be helpful. It eased the tension quite a bit and made my headaches go away. I usually drank two or three cups a day while awaiting the final outcome," she said.

A unique lottery system was devised by the CPA firm that did the re-count and by the Clearfield City Recorder, Richard B. Waite. Monson won the right to make the first call on the coin toss, and chose the "heads" side. This left Ms. Layton with the tail end of things, quite literally. "I think I must have drunk five cups of peppermint tea the rest of that day," she stated with a laugh.

The coin toss occurred the next morning in the council room of the Clearfield City offices. Waite wanted to use a coin bigger than the size of a silver dollar so everyone could see it plainly enough. So he chose his 1974 BYU National Football Champion commemorative coin for the flipping contest. On the heads side was BYU Coach LaVell Edwards, while the tails side included a large *Y*.

It was a small but historic moment the morning of Tuesday, November 14, as Waite's special coin went up in the air a few feet and then flopped down onto the carpet. There were signs of relief, a groan of disappointment for Monson, and an exclaimed noise of elation from Ms. Layton. "From the looks of things," she said with a satisfied smile, "I'm going to be on the city council for a couple more years."

WINNING TEA

1 pint water

2 tbsp. dried peppermint leaves

Boil the water, then add the leaves. Stir and cover with a lid. Set aside to steep for 20 minutes. Strain and sweeten with a pinch of brown sugar, if necessary. Drink warm between meals several times throughout the day.

NEURALGIA

The Remedies of a Medical Herbalist

DESCRIPTION

Neuralgia is a condition in which the facial nerves become inflamed to varying degrees. The cause is usually brought on by exposure to chills and drafts. A person becomes more susceptible to neuralgia when his or her immune system is run down. The pain from the affected nerve, known as neuralgia, is severe and localized along the path of the nerve itself. The skin is frequently hypersensitive, with the slightest light touch producing immediate discomfort.

Two for Tea

Annie Goodhart has lived in London, England, for most of her life. In 1995 she was 31 years of age. She studied botanical medicine at the School of Phytotherapy in Sussex for five years before becoming certified as a medical herbalist. She practices her healing craft in the heart of the London business district.

One of her clients, a prominent financier with the Bank of England, came to her sometime in 1994 suffering from excruciating neuralgia in the left side of his face and neck.

She made a tea from two herbs, St. Johnswort and lavender, and gave him some of that to drink while he was there. He reported feeling better within minutes of taking it. She showed him how to make it and encouraged him to continue taking it for a week or more. He did so, and his condition cleared up completely and had not returned as of this writing (late November 1995).

ANNIE'S FORMULA FOR PAIN RELIEF

1¹/₄ pints water

2 tsp. St. Johnswort, cut and dried

1 tsp. lavender flowers, cut and dried

Put the dried herbs in the bottom of a fruit jar or small tea kettle. Boil the water and pour it over them. Cover with a lid and steep for 15 minutes. Strain into another container, seal with a lid, and store excess in a cool place but *not* necessarily the refrigerator. Reheat what is intended to be used. Slowly sip the moderately *hot* tea from a cup or mug.

Furthermore, an embrocation can be made from the same tea and applied directly to the surface of the skin. The tea needs to be hot enough for this to work. Use some ice tongs to soak a clean washcloth in the tea solution; wring out the excess by pressing the cloth against the sides of the pot with the back of a wooden spoon. Fold into a neat little square with the tongs and apply directly to the site of pain and cover with a folded dry hand towel to keep as much heat in for the longest time possible.

Ms. Goodhart said she never knew this remedy to fail in relieving the worst types of pain, including sciatica, toothache, migraines, muscle pains, and so forth.

NIGHT SWEATS

Something to Help You Sleep Dry

DESCRIPTION

A night sweat is profuse perspiration during sleep. It occurs in cases of pulmonary tuberculosis, acquired immune deficiency syndrome (AIDS), and other chronic debilitating affections with low-grade fever.

Ancient Latin Remedy

Some years ago I was passing through Rome, Italy, on some research business elsewhere in Europe. I had about six hours between connecting flights, so I visited the Vatican Library for a few hours. It rates among scholars as one of the great libraries of the entire world. It is and has always been, first and foremost, a manuscript library. There are an estimated 50,000+ manuscripts housed in its vast collections; some of these date back *to before the time of Christ*. The entire manuscript inventory is divided between closed and open collections.

An assistant prefect or associate director (usually a Jesuit scholar) by the name of Father Zeladiana brought out several very brittle and considerably yellowed parchments dating back to A.D. 650. Because of their very old and delicate condition they had been carefully preserved between sheets of rigid plastic. On them were written in ancient Latin several herbal formulas that were once used to treat some of the earliest popes of the Roman Catholic Church.

Because I couldn't read a word of Latin, Father Zeladiana had another Jesuit priest working in the library who spoke pretty good English assist me in translating what was written on both documents. This other fellow's name was Father Leone Chiaramonti, S.J. He read for me slowly as I scribbled out on my yellow legal pad the English translation to the first document.

It concerned a remedy devised by one Vatican doctor for Pope Felix IV, who presided over the church from July 526 to September 530. The document that Father Chiaramonti was reading for me told about this particular pope being subject to night sweats during a bout with fever. Different remedies were tried by several attending physicians, but nothing seemed to work.

Then one of these doctors developed an herbal formula which was made into a tea and given to the ailing pope in copious amounts. The night sweats ceased almost immediately, and the pope became better after that. No specific amounts were mentioned in the manuscript sheet, only the formula preparation in itself.

TEA FOR THE POPE

1³/₄ pints water

1 handful sage leaves

1/2 handful rosemary leaves

1/2 handful boneset

Boil the water. Add the sage and rosemary first. Cover and simmer over low heat for 3 minutes. Uncover and add the boneset; cover again and set aside to steep until cold. Strain and drink 2 cups every 4 to 6 hours until perspiration ceases.

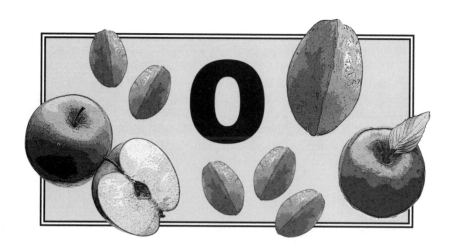

<u>OBESITY</u>

How a Secret Herbal Brew Enabled One Overweight Catholic Pope to Shed Many Unwanted Pounds

DESCRIPTION

If the reader hasn't looked at the preceding entry of NIGHT SWEATS, he or she is encouraged to do so, because this is a continuation of my brief visit to the Vatican Library in Rome, Italy, some years ago. At that time I had the assistance of Father Leone Chiaramonti, S.J., then a member of the library staff, who translated for me into English some heretofore unknown herbal remedies mentioned in a couple of very ancient-looking but carefully preserved handwritten Latin manuscript sheets.

Secret Weight Loss Formula of the Popes

Boniface II was elected pope on September 17, A.D. 530, following the death of his predecessor Felix IV. Boniface had served the Roman Church from his early youth. During the reign of Felix IV, he was archdeacon and a personage of considerable influence with the ecclesiastical and civil authorities.

His elevation to the papacy is one of the most remarkable in the history of the church. It offered an unquestionable example of the

245

nomination of a pope by his predecessor, without even the formality of an election (as it has always been done for many centuries).

Felix IV, approaching death and fearing a contest for the papacy between Roman and Gothic factions, gathered around him several of his most trusted clergy and a number of Roman Senators and patricians who happened to be nearby. In their presence, he solemnly conferred on archdeacon the pallium of papal sovereignty, proclaiming him his successor and threatening with excommunication anyone who refused to recognize and obey Boniface as the validly chosen pope.

Upon Felix's death, Boniface assumed succession, but nearly all of the Roman priests, probably 60 out of roughly 70, refused to accept him and elected Dioscorus. Both popes were consecrated on September 22, A.D. 530, Boniface in the basilica of Julius and Dioscorus in the Lateran. Fortunately it endured but 22 days, for Dioscorus died on October 14, quite suddenly of symptoms closely resembling those of a classic heart attack. He was almost 40 pounds overweight at the time of his unexpected demise.

This left Boniface unchallenged and in total possession of the papacy. But, like many of his predecessors before and after him, he loved to eat good food and drink fine wines. However, the amount of physical exercise he got each day was quite minimal. Therefore, his nearly 50 pounds of excess weight carried around on a body only five feet five inches high posed a great health risk for him.

Vatican court doctors were understandably alarmed by his periodic bouts of belabored breathing and occasional chest pains. So they worked hard to come up with a natural solution to this added burden of weight. They devised an herbal combination to be made into a tea, which they had Boniface II drink *seven times* a day. The ancient parchment on which all of this was written in old Latin and kindly translated for me by Father Chiaramonti, S.J., clearly mentioned, however, that this formula was *carefully administered* to His Holiness the Pope *under medical supervision*. The reason for this was apparently because of the Alexandrian senna present in the mixture, which has strong purgative effects when taken alone. No problems with the formula were cited anywhere in the extremely weathered manuscript, except to say that "the physicians watched over the Holy Father during the period of his medicine." This should serve as a cautionary note to those wishing to try this simple remedy for themselves in the hopes of losing weight.

What the manuscript *did not* revel was just how much weight the pope actually lost. But it seems that the formula worked pretty well, because court doctors noted that "His Holiness is breathing much better, complains no more of chest pains, is more nimble in step and cheerful in spirit" and also "is not so large around his middle" anymore. Since the time I was in Rome many years ago, I have recommended this tea to several dozen friends and colleagues who were troubled with varying degrees of obesity and had tried everything in their power to lose some weight, most often unsuccessfully. Once I convinced them to give the tea a try, many reported losing more weight than expected; only a few complained about its not working. But upon carefully questioning the complainers, I soon discovered that they had not been taking it *seven times a day* as the manuscript suggested to be done. Those for whom it always worked took it faithfully and regularly without fail. How much weight do you intend losing? Will you be willing to try it faithfully or embrace it only half-heartedly? Ultimately, your physical shape will determine just how much effort and consistency you put into drinking the tea.

THE PAPACY'S WEIGHT-LOSS TEA

7 parts dandelion root and leaves

5 parts burdock root and leaves

17 parts peppermint leaves

15 parts alder buckthorn bark

10 Alexandrian senna leaflets and fruit

9 parts yarrow herb

9 parts witch grass (also known as couch grass, dog grass, quack grass; Agropyron repens)

1 kettle full of water

The original manuscript parchment listed these herbs only by "parts" and nothing else. In trying to convert this to something that makes sense for modern applications, I came up with teaspoons—two parts of the Latin would be equivalent to one level teaspoon of the modern rendering. Also, a "kettle full of water" would be about $1^1/_2$ gallons.

The page that Father Chiaramonti, S.J. (Society of Jesus or Jesuit) translated for my benefit said just to "boil everything until half the liquid remains in the kettle." I took this to mean that *all* of the ingredients were added at once, and the kettle was covered over with a lid and simmered on low heat for about an hour or until approximately half the water remained.

It was then strained, cooled, and taken in small glassfuls throughout the day. No further attention was devoted as to *when* was the best time to take it. But based on the information given to me by some of those who've tried it in past years and lost weight, the tea should be taken following a meal or even a piece of bread. When it is taken on an empty stomach there have been occasional reports of some gastrointestinal discomforts from it. So to avoid such unpleasantries, I advise that something be eaten with each *small* (6 fluid ounce) glassful.

Also readers should be aware that *any* herbs known for their purgative, laxative, or detoxifying properties are going to flush *some* minerals and vitamins out of the body. So it is *very important* that anyone drinking such a tea take a high-potency vitamin-mineral complex each day (four tablets with one meal of the day).

Overall, this ancient formula is quite safe, unbelievably effective, and gentle to use. If it worked for some of the old Catholic Fathers in bygone centuries in helping them shed some of their corpulency, then it should do justice to some of your unwanted pounds.

OSTEOPOROSIS

also:

OVARIAN BLEEDING

PARKINSON'S DISEASE

PEPTIC ULCER

PREMENSTRUAL SYNDROME (PMS)

PROSTATE DISORDERS

PSORIASIS

Sunrise Breakfast Shake: "Miracle" Health Drink in a Glass

DESCRIPTION

The seven disorders listed above, while obviously different in certain ways, also share some very common and basic attributes. These would include pain, inflammation, swelling, some bleeding, infection, weak immunity, and nutritional deficiencies. It is my opinion, based on the sound research information to be presented here, that each of these problems can be adequately treated with the appropriate food, herbs, and nutrients to be mentioned in this section.

Something About the Work I Do

For two decades, I have been the sole Director of the Anthropological Research Center in Salt Lake City, Utah. My staff and I conduct research that specifically applies to the medical and nutritional sides of human culture, both past and present. We also look into a number of other social aspects related to humankind that don't always connect with remedies or diet.

Our work is both of a private and a public nature. Almost all the national and foreign research expeditions I have been on in the past two and a half decades have been strictly for the purpose of gathering valuable data for most of my health books, newsletters, articles, and lectures. A number of different companies in the gigantic health food supplement industry have solicited our services over the years for different reasons. In some instances they've wanted information on a particular botanical or nutrient, which we provide them. At other times they may want literature written on a specific item and come to us because they know it will be correct and proper. And every so often, clients will approach us asking our research center to help them develop a specific product they have in mind, based on the details they've given us.

The public side of the many services we've rendered come in several different forms. First, there are those doctors scattered from coast to coast who may write or call wanting more data on something some of their patients might be taking with which they're not too familiar. And, every now and again, a city, state, or federal agency might initiate contact to know if an herb or herbal product is deemed relatively safe for public consumption. Or they may ask us to explain to them how one or several remedies fit into the culture of a particular ethnic group.

But, by far, the biggest share of public service we render is to people such as yourself all over America, in Canada and Mexico, as well as in Europe and other parts of the world where my books have become best-sellers. The volume of mail received into this research center on a monthly basis is overwhelming. Individuals from all walks of life write wanting to know what is best for their own health problems. We try to help them but within very carefully defined guidelines so that at *no time* are we ever guilty of prescribing without a medical license.

This, then, is a short summary of the many unique services we try to provide to those who make contact with us at any given time. However in the process of assisting others, we sometimes are asked to approach a specific assignment from a perspective that jointly involves food, herbs, and nutrients. In order to meet any of these wonderful challenges successfully, we must then conduct extensive research that will lead to a satisfactory solution for our clients, incorporating all three sources into whatever we come up with for them.

Because of confidentiality agreements that we have with nearly all our health care and supplement clients, we can never divulge specific identities, their geographical locations, or the personal terms of the work performed for them. But, in a very broad and general sense I and my staff are at liberty to discuss a number of elements that are basic to a project just completed. This is what I propose doing here, while at the same time respecting the privacy of a particular client.

Suffice it to say, a while back I was contacted by an alternative health care organization that wanted us to develop for them a way in which they could give their clients basic nutrition and medicine *at one time* without repeated efforts later in the day. And they wanted it *versatile enough* so that any number of different foods, botanicals, or nutritional supplements could be added for *specific* problems. In other words, they were looking for a *universal* way of administering things, but so flexible that it could be customized to the individual needs and wants of their patients.

Morning Nutrition Is Where It's at

Working within the parameters given us, we spent a great deal of time, effort, and funds researching the matter. The first thing we realized was that *the morning* was the most *ideal* time for a person to be taking food, herbs, and vitamins/minerals. The second thing we discovered was the easiest and most convenient form in which to take such things would be a *drink shake* of some kind. We opted for something more vegetable-based than fruit-derived, because of the prevailing belief that minerals in the former are more important than sweet carbohydrates in the latter. Also, a vegetable-based shake could be taken by both diabetics and hypoglycemics, whereas anything fruit-derived couldn't be.

Further research enabled us to build on the base we had already established. We evaluated dozens of different things and came up with a small but significant group of items that we felt best represented a good cross-section of what the body needs on a daily basis. These things were to be *added* to the shake and then consumed by our client's patients. But the formula was flexible enough to permit our client to add a *few other* natural supplements (in powder or liquid forms) that they felt would be necessary for the *individual* needs of each patient receiving this shake.

We delivered the finished program to our client, who was delighted with it. This large alternative health care facility then began using it with several hundred of their patients, who had a variety of problems. In nearly every instance, patients' conditions improved remarkably with our formula drink and our client's own inclusion of other natural substances based on individual patient needs.

After receiving from our client the results of this one-year "testing," I asked for and received their permission to incorporate some of the data in this book. The only understood proviso was that I respect the privacy agreement between us. And now, after having said all this, let me get into the heart of the program itself.

The Basics of My "Wonder Tonic"

My "miracle health drink," as it has been called by a number of different people on both sides of the project equation, uses a specific vegetable protein as the base to work from. I can't give out the mixture we developed for our client, but I can offer a close equivalent to it in the marketplace. Readers are advised to look for Nature's fat-free Vegetable Protein All Natural Instant Powder Mix in their local health food stores or nutrition centers. This company has been around since 1926 and is one of the most respected of its kind in the giant health food industry. Their protein sources for the mix include soy, sprouted barley, sesame meal, pea, and rice. Their fiber mix includes corn, apple, and pea. Their enzymes are derived from papaya and pineapple. With the exception of five items that we included in our drink formula, this Naturade product very closely approximates what I came up with for my unnamed client. An average of 4 teaspoons in $2^1/_2$ cups (20 ounces) of liquid is suggested.

The next ingredient is goat milk, simply because it is easier to digest than regular cow's milk. I highly recommend a *powdered* goat milk for this. It doesn't need to be refrigerated, but can be stored for up to two months in a cool, dry place. It can be taken with you wherever you go and is easy to mix. Add 9 level tablespoons of the powder to the $2^1/_2$ cups of water previously mentioned. Stir thoroughly or blend in a Vita-Mix machine or an equivalent food machine with the vegetable protein powder to make a smooth, even-textured drink.

Beets and chlorophyll form the next part of my "wonder tonic" drink. The best source for both is Pines International of Lawrence, Kansas. They make the best organic beet root and wheat grass juice concentrates in the industry. (See Product Appendix for more information.) Add one level teaspoon each of beet powder and wheat grass powder to the aforementioned nutrition shake.

Follow this with one-half teaspoon each of American ginseng extract, Swedish bitters, and Kyolic Garlic. These liquid extracts can be obtained from local health food stores or from the manufacturers themselves:

American ginseng
Vermont Ginseng Products
Waterbury, VT 05676 (800-270-0007)
Swedish bitters
NatureWorks
207 E. 94th St.
New York, NY 10128 (800-843-9535)

Kyolic Garlic
Wakunaga of America
23501 Madero
Mission Viejo, CA 92691 (800-421-2998)

Finally, add one-quarter banana (peeled and cut) to the breakfast shake and blend for one minute at top speed until everything is creamy smooth. Drink this for your breakfast or with your morning meal. Other things can be added on an "as needed" basis for any individual health problems cited in this section.

Osteoporosis. The patients that this anonymous health care facility treated with this formula mix added 2,000 mg. of calcium powder and 1,400 mg. of magnesium powder to it. In the event that neither is available to you in powders, an equivalent amount can be obtained by crushing up some tablets of each. Another alternative is adding 1 level tablespoon of blackstrap molasses. But if this poses some risk to diabetics or hypoglycemics, then use 1 level teaspoon of powdered brewer's yeast instead. The shake was given every morning for two months and then reduced to three times weekly, given every other day.

Ovarian Problems. Female patients being treated by my client for different ovarian disorders were given this shake with 20 drops of fluid extract of birthwort and $1/2$ teaspoon alfalfa powder added to it. At other times, $1/2$ cup red clover tea and 20 drops of fluid extract of black cohosh were added instead. In the event of serious infections, $1/2$ teaspoon powdered goldenseal root or echinacea along with 5,000 mg. of vitamin C crystals were substituted. Patients were encouraged to drink this on a fairly regular basis.

Parkinson's Disease. Older patients who suffered from this shaking palsy were instructed by their attending doctors to drink my "wonder tonic," but with these additions: $1/2$ level teaspoon each of calcium and magnesium powders; 1 teaspoon of flaxseed or evening primrose oils; 1 teaspoon of lecithin (liquid or granules); $1/2$ teaspoon amino acid complex powder; and $1/4$ teaspoon brewer's yeast. This disorder is quite common—even U.S. Attorney General Janet Reno stated in late November 1995 that she had been diagnosed with Parkinson's.

Peptic Ulcer. Many of those who came to the aforementioned facility were treated for peptic ulcers. Nearly all of them had been longtime users of Zantac or Tagamet, the two most commonly prescribed medications for this problem, or they relied heavily upon "the pink, runny stuff" (Pepto-Bismol) for relief. But based on the research of a brash young Australian doctor from Perth, doctors decided to use antibiotics and bismuth instead. However, they wisely substituted liquid Kyolic Garlic (2 teaspoons), liquid vitamin C (1 tablespoon), and $1/2$ teaspoon powdered goldenseal root, all of which were mixed in with the regular ingredients of the shake. Patients were told to drink a cup in the morning and again at night with meals. Many reported considerable improvement within a week of beginning treatment.

Premenstrual Syndrome (PMS). Women experiencing PMS were advised to drink *two* cups of my "sunrise breakfast shake" in the morning and again at night, if necessary. But to every two cups made in the blender the following additional items were added: 1 teaspoon each of calcium and magnesium (or the equivalent of 1,500 mg. apiece); 1 teaspoon vitamin B-complex powder (or the equivalent derived from some crushed tablets of the same); and 25 drops of fluid extract of black cohosh.

Prostate Disorders. It is now know that one in every five American males has some form of prostate trouble. Men who were treated at the previously cited alternative health care facility took the shake every day with these other items included: $1/2$ teaspoon zinc powder; $1/2$ teaspoon raw bee pollen; $1/2$ teaspoon beta-carotene powder; and $1/2$ teaspoon raw animal glandular (prostate) powder. Sometimes $1/2$ teaspoon desiccated liver powder was put in just for good measure.

Psoriasis. It is interesting that while the majority of those patients treated at my former client's facility were mature adults, a fair number of teenagers and college-age kids were seen by doctors for this hereditary skin disorder. With great relish, they immediately took to the morning shake idea, to which was added 1 teaspoon cold-pressed flaxseed oil, 1 teaspoon emulsified vitamin A, and 1 teaspoon powdered vitamin B-complex (made from crushed tablets).

Adjustments May Be Necessary

Among the data results of a yearlong trial study with my nourishing drink came the realization that the suggested measurements for some of the ingredients might have to readjusted up or down according to what else was added. In some cases, the water had to be slightly increased or more banana included to improve the flavor (if bitter or bad-tasting substances were called for in specific problems).

But, like everything else that's tried for the first time, it became better in terms of flavor and consistency once all the kinks were out of it.

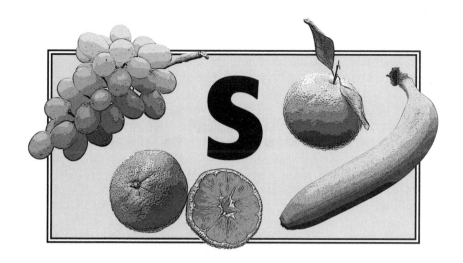

SHINGLES

(see Herpes Zoster)

SMOKING HABIT

Licorice-Ginger Tea Combo Helps Break the Nicotine Habit

DESCRIPTION

Licorice is a perennial that prefers temperate climate zones in which to grow. It can be either an herb or a type of shrub, 3 to 7 feet high, with a long, cylindrical, branched, flexible, burrowing rootstock. The underground stems are horizontal creeping and attain 5 to 6 feet in length, with buds that send up stems in the second year. The leaves are alternate, pinnate, with 9 to 17 ovate yellow-green leaflets, long, and with a sticky underside to them. Flowers appear as erect, axillary, long-stalked spikes 4 to 6 inches long. They are pealike, lavender to purple in hue, and $1/2$ inch in length.

The French Foreign Legion has issued rations of licorice root to some of its desert units to help allay intense thirst where water is in short supply. Tea is made from chunks of the peeled, dried, coarsely cut root and put into soldiers' canteens; they then take periodic swigs of this throughout the day and are able to get by with less water. Some French doctors still rely on licorice root to treat dry coughs, bronchial laryngitis, urinary irritation, and painful diarrhea.

Common ginger is an erect perennial herb with thick tuberous underground stems or rhizomes from which another stem (the aerial) grows up to about 1 yard high. It is extensively cultivated in the tropics.

In Tonga, a species of ginger root *(Zingiber zerumbet)* is used for a variety of ailments of the mouth, including *pala ngutu* (mouth sores), *pale fefie* (oral thrush), *kiaotolu nifo* (swollen gums), and for *kahi* (internal blockage). In Samoa, ginger root is used in a special mix with another herb *(Homalanthus acuminatus)* to treat *tulita* (abdominal distress). In all of these uses, ginger root is used in the form of a tea.

Freedom from Nicotine Fits

A certain Jane Doe (who requested anonymity), in Peoria, Illinois, age 33 and with a promising career in television communications, took up smoking about seven years ago for a very strange reason. "One of my other identities," she told me by telephone, "said that smoking would help to relax me. So I started smoking Virginia Slims and was surprised at how much it helped relieve tension on the job."

But after being told by her physician that she ran the risk of incurring breast cancer if she continued smoking, Jane Doe opted to quit. However, that was easier said than done. "I tried different methods of quitting, but always ended going back for more cigarettes," she acknowledged. She finally managed to find something, though, that was very promising in helping her to kick the smoking habit so she wouldn't get any more nicotine fits.

But the *way* in which she realized a solution that actually worked for her is rather bizarre to say the least. Ms. Doe attributed the herbal tea combination she used to "another of my many identities." My informant, you must understand, was diagnosed some years ago by psychiatrists as having Multiple Personality Disorder (MPD), now called Dissociative Identity Disorder (DID). This Jane Doe claims to have 21 "different identities working in my behalf."

Needless to say, the remedy she used *worked* in spite of its somewhat questionable source of origin. She was "told" to make a tea using licorice and ginger roots and to *sip a warm cup* every time a nicotine craving came over her. Within two weeks of doing this her smoking habit had completely disappeared.

As we were finishing our long-distance phone call, Ms. Doe's voice suddenly changed to a very different tone and I found myself speaking to someone else claiming another first name. I quickly ended the conversation and hung up.

ANTI-SMOKING TEA

1 pint water
1 tsp. licorice root
$^1/_2$ tsp. ginger root
$^1/_4$ tsp. fenugreek seed

Boil the water. Then add the roots and seeds. Cover with a lid, lower heat, and simmer for 10 minutes. Then set aside and steep for 15 minutes. Strain and refrigerate. Reheat until somewhat warm before drinking.

STOMACH ULCERS

(see Peptic Ulcer)

STRESS

Two-Mint Tea Alleviates Fear of Ghosts for Female Mortician

DESCRIPTION

"Enrollment is at an all-time high," Gordon Bigelow told me by telephone from his office in Brunswick, Maine, in late November 1995. He is the executive director of the American Board of Funeral Service Education, which tracks statistics at the nation's 42 colleges of mortuary science.

And the would-be undertakers are getting older, he noted, with an average age now of around 27 instead of in the lower twenties as in former times. Besides this, many are choosing funeral services as their second or third career, after being laid off or experiencing "job burnout" elsewhere. In 1995, more than 3,150 students were enrolled; this is up from 2,200 in 1991—36 percent are women, up from 9 percent a decade ago.

The U.S. Labor Department predicts that the employment opportunities in mortuary science are "quite excellent" through the year 2005. The explanation given for this assessment is that "death has a steady growth rate," requiring more undertakers.

Tucking in the Corpses

Sue Allison goes through the same routine every night during her $9,000, 12-month internship at the San Francisco College of Mortuary Science. Over the phone she explained what she had to do during the Thanksgiving week of November 1995.

"Every night before I leave, I make sure all the corpses are neatly tucked away in their respective boxes," she stated in very straightforward honesty. "I check all of them, and straighten a tie if it needs it or fix a lock of hair before telling them all good night." She described her daily attire as always being some kind of a "black dress." "Black is the 'in' thing out here," she continued. "They won't even let you near the bodies unless you're wearing black. It's all quite formal you know."

She described for me in great detail the long days and nights of lifting bodies into unmarked vans, injecting embalming fluid into veins, trimming toenails on corpses, and talking to grieving families who come to the school's low-cost student-run mortuary, the only such establishment in the nation.

"I know this sounds kind of crazy," she said in a halting tone of voice. "But I actually love what I do. For me and many other of my student friends out here, it's like every day is Halloween. I mean, it's exciting and challenging. I can't think of anything I'd rather be doing more right now than working with dead bodies. *It's fun!"*

Peppermint and Lemon Balm

But under more careful questioning, Sue admitted that when she first came to the school, "the corpses really freaked me out at first. Especially when it came my turn to 'tuck them in' as it's called out here when we have to check them in their caskets. I was under a lot of stress in the beginning and actually broke out in hives because of it."

She went to a San Francisco herb shop on the famous Market Street and was given an anti-stress tea formula, which she started taking. "Right away, I could begin to feel its effects on my nervous system," she confided. "I mean, it was as if all my fears suddenly left me. After just a couple of days of drinking the tea, I felt totally relaxed. Now, I look forward to taking my turn to 'tuck in the corpses.'" After a moment's pause, she added, "I don't know if this means anything, but I rent a bedroom apartment in a local funeral home. It just seems more appropriate for the kind of education I'm getting."

STRESS-FREE TEA

4¹/₂ cups water

2 tbsp. lemon balm leaves

1 tbsp. peppermint leaves

1 tsp. lemon juice

Boil the water. Add the herbs, stir thoroughly, and cover with lid. Then set aside and steep for 25 minutes. Strain and stir in lemon juice before refrigerating. Reheat only the amount desired and drink lukewarm on an empty stomach several times daily.

STROKE

Rehabilitation Tea Formula for Restoration of Bodily Functions

DESCRIPTION

Stroke is the third leading health problem in America today, right behind heart disease and cancer. According to figures supplied by the National Stroke Association, an estimated three quarters of a million people every year suffer a stroke somewhere in America. Of this number nearly one quarter of a million die. Stroke also happens to be the leading cause of adult disability in the country. In fact, there are almost three million people in the nation right now living with the aftereffects of stroke.

A stroke can best be described as an immediate disruption in the flow of blood that supplies life-supporting oxygen and nutrients to the brain. Once deprived of blood for even the briefest moment of time, the affected brain cells are either damaged or just die. When this happens bodily functions previously controlled by those damaged or dead brain cells are quickly impaired. The duration of impairment depends, of course, upon the length of blood deprivation to that portion of brain tissue adversely affected by a stroke.

A stroke isn't just something that happens very quickly. Rather it is a slow and continuous build-up of problems over a long period of time. Fat, cholesterol, and other substances that clog heart and neck arteries produce a narrowing of artery walls and a significant reduction in blood flow through the body. A stroke is the climax of such extreme blood constriction.

Partial Imprisonment Within Yourself

The most common symptom of a stroke is paralysis on one side of the body. The left hemisphere of the brain controls right-body functions, while the right hemisphere is in charge of left-body functions. Ordinarily a stroke occurs only in one side of the brain; when this happens only certain portions of bodily functions are lost.

To best understand how terrible a stroke can be to someone unfortunate enough to experience it, conduct this simple mental experiment on yourself. Imagine that you are wearing a straight jacket, but with your left arm outside hanging free. Then picture a 25-pound iron ball chained to your right ankle. Finally, think of how numb the right side of your jaw and lips would be if a dentist injected it with a large dose of Novocain. There you have a mental image that closely approximates what a right-side stroke paralysis would be.

The gifted choreographer Agnes de Mille, when alive, suffered a massive stroke many years ago in the left hemisphere of the brain that paralyzed the entire right side of her body. In describing how it felt, she noted some time later, "Half of me was imprisoned in the other half of my body. My dead side seemed unaccountably heavy, gigantically heavy and restrained with bonds that seemed to be made of iron, cement, or wood. When I rolled in my bed and tried to get onto my right, or dead, side, I rolled against a dyke of unfeeling matter which I lacked the strength to go over or rise against."

Besides the paralysis, Ms. de Mille also had to put up with a nerve disorder that involved jerky uncontrolled movement. She recalled this additional agony in these words: "There were, at times, irrational and insane jerkings which I wasn't aware of. My hand would fly out and encounter . . . well . . . whatever there was to encounter. And my attempts in training that right hand to do the most primitive bidding was like training a wild animal. It didn't seem like my hand at all. In fact, it wasn't anybody's hand. It could have been the hind leg of a donkey, for that matter."

Stroke Rehabilitation Tea

Stroke rehabilitation requires a multifaceted approach and involves the teamwork of many care providers. Physical and occupational therapies form the backbone of this program to get a stroke survivor up and moving around again. Speech and language therapies follow next to help a stroke patient speak and hear again and regain whatever mental understanding may have been temporarily lost. Next comes some form of psychological counseling, which enables the patient to deal with his or her post-stroke depression and other emotional issues frequently associated with this problem. The services of recreational therapists and vocational counselors also come into play here to help the stroke survivor explore how he or she will best utilize his or her time upon returning home. Then comes the challenge of being able to put it all together again with the support of friends and loved ones.

During 1994 my writing talents were solicited by Dr. David Steenblock, the director of the Steenblock Institute for Stroke Recovery in Mission Viejo, California. He wanted me to be the co-author of a book with him on the subject of stroke. Considerable time and resources were involved in this most worthy project. I spent some weeks at his private research center and library in the hills of San Clemente, with a lovely view overlooking the white sandy beach and Pacific Ocean some distance below. Many hours were spent every day in what I now refer to as a "crash course" in familiarizing myself with just about every aspect of stroke. Never had I plunged myself into such an intense learning experience on a single topic as this. By the time I was finished, I probably knew more about stroke than most doctors do.

One of the things that was necessary for me to become involved with to a degree were some of Dr. Steenblock's stroke patients, who were being treated on a daily basis at his clinic. I had free access to their medical records and permission from Dr. Steenblock himself to interview as many of them as I wanted. Most of those whom I interviewed at great length were very cooperative. They gave me a tremendous insight into stroke that I never had before.

My colleague, David, wanted one section of the book to include a list of those particular botanicals that would be especially efficacious in the recovery program of potential stroke victims. Once I understood all aspects of the disability I was dealing with, I was able to formulate the appropriate herbal therapy for it. Unfortunately for both of us, the project languished even though I had found a publisher for our impending book. Due to some serious setbacks and misfortunes experienced at David's clinic, the book eventually "withered on the vine," as the old adage goes.

During various public lectures at a number of health conventions given around the country during 1995, I would make frequent references to a Rehabilitation Tea that I had formulated especially for stroke victims. Close to a dozen different individuals approached me and inquired more about this herbal combination. They were anxious to try it on some of their friends or relatives who had become victims of stroke.

A total of 11 people were given the tea per my instructions by their respective caregivers. Of that number, four subjects had been suffering stroke for six months or longer, while the rest had been disabled for shorter periods. Two had been crippled between four and five months, and the other five for *less than a month!* (I emphasize this last time in italics, because it played a very significant factor in patient recoveries.)

The tea was administered three times daily between meals for periods lasting anywhere from six weeks to almost three months. Each of those caregivers who agreed to participate in this informal study diligently reported the progress of their stroke victims to me in writing or by phone. Not surprisingly, those who had strokes of *under 30 days* demonstrated the *greastest recovery* from paralysis, but (and this is important to remember) *in conjunction* with other modalities of therapy. The rule of thumb here seems to have been that *the longer* the time elapsed since the stroke, *the less* evidence there was of regaining physical functions.

John's Stroke Rehabilitation Tea

1 quart spring or mineral water

1 tsp. fenugreek seed

1 tsp. celery with leaves, finely cut

1 tsp. carrot with leafy top (if possible), finely cut

1 tsp. red pontiac potato peeling, grated (organic)

1 tsp. dark-brown vanilla pods, crushed

1 tsp. lemon balm

1 tsp. peppermint leaves

1 tsp. spearmint leaves

1 tsp. catnip

Boil the water. Then add the next five ingredients, from the fenugreek seeds to the vanilla pods. Cover with lid and simmer on reduced heat for 20 minutes. Then add the last four mint herbs. Cover again, set aside, and steep for 20 more minutes. *DO NOT strain!* Keep only at room temperature; *don't refrigerate.*

The caregivers should see that a stroke victim gets three glasses daily between meals. Only then may the tea be strained, reheated until warm before administering. The potted tea can be kept in a cool, dry place for no more than 24 hours.

The reason this tea appears to work so well in *early* cases of stroke that are no more than several weeks old is that it seems to deliver to the brain those nutrients and other chemical compounds that *increase* oxygen in the blood, and it promotes more active circulation to those areas of the brain that have been damaged by stroke.

SWEATING

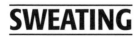

(see Night Sweats)

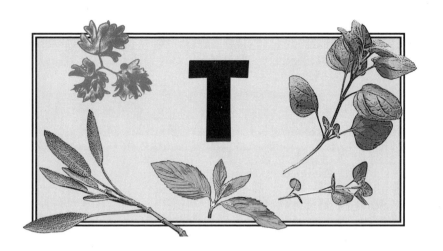

THYROID DYSFUNCTION

Retired Nurse Finds My Juice Recommendations Very Helpful

DESCRIPTION

Every month the Anthropological Research Center in Salt Lake City, Utah, receives on the average about 715 pieces of mail from people who have bought one or several of my different health encyclopedias. The majority of them contain rave reviews about the books I write.

Typical of such correspondence is one I recently received, dated November 26, 1995, from a retired licensed practical nurse named Frieda Hein, who resides in Oak Park, Illinois. A portion of her letter is excerpted here with her kind consent.

John Heinerman
Salt Lake City, UT

Dear Dr. Heinerman:

I bought your book "The Encyclopedia of Healing Juices" and I think it's the most helpful health book there is. I have lots of other health books in my small library, but none of them stack up to yours.

I have a small lay-evangelism and health school and I am a nutritionist, so I know a lot of people who would want your book.

Keep up the good work. You're helping more people than you know about. God bless you!

/s/ Frieda Hein

Oak Park, IL 60302

Thyroid Problems Disappear with my Juice Recommendations

Since she had included a phone number, I decided to call her on Wednesday, November 29, 1995. We had a lovely chat. Frieda informed me that she had been practicing nursing for 35 of her 72 years of life. "I saw too much corruption within the medical profession," she said, "and I decided to do something about it. So I started reading all the health books I could get my hands on and became knowledgeable in many things that they never taught us in nursing school when I was a student going there." She then named several health titles published decades ago by such well-known authors as Bernard Jensen, Adelle Davis, and Bernard MacFadden.

"I had been suffering from thyroid problems, weak adrenal glands, and a weak heart," she mentioned. "But mostly it's been a weak, inactive thyroid that has caused a lot of my problems. Then I ordered your *Healing Juices* book from the publisher and began reading it. I decided to try some of your recommendations."

She said that an inability to get a good night's rest was one of the things her doctors linked to her thyroid dysfunction.

"I read in your book . . . wait a minute while I hunt it down," she continued. About a minute passed before she returned to the phone. "Here it is on page 120 of your book *[Heinerman's Encyclopedia of Healing Juices]*." And then she proceeded to read aloud to me the two sentences of importance to her.

> **Insomnia.** The consumption of carbohydrate-rich foods towards bedtime will, quite often, induce sleep very soon thereafter. A little date-fig juice may be the perfect night-cap an insomniac is after, provided he or she doesn't have blood-sugar problems.

"I want you to know what happened when I did this," she continued. "I took just one date and one fig and mixed them up in my food blender with a little water and drank that before going to bed. Ordinarily, I would be awake half the night, tossing and turning. But after I drank this half cup of that date-fig juice, I slept like a baby. Why, I didn't wake up until 10:00 o'clock the next morning. I never slept so long in my life. I felt as if I had just been given a new lease on life!"

Then she made reference to the wonderful things she had experienced using my apple-spinach combination as recommended on page 9 of my book. "Another of my difficulties has been with my digestive system," she said. "Doctors seem to think it's more connected with my thyroid problems than with any indigestion. I took a cup of the apple-spinach juice in the afternoon and, right away, felt very, very good. I was astonished at just how quickly the effect worked so well on me and quite amazed at how delicious it tasted."

She explained what my grape-raisin juice combination mentioned on page 141 did for her energy levels. "I took a little bit [exact amount unspecified] and felt an energy surge almost immediately. It was like being plugged into a wall outlet and suddenly coming alive with food current," she added.

Frieda has been teaching weekly classes on health and nutrition for a number of years. Anywhere from 10 to 20 older women get together for this wonderful educational experience. She feels a tremendous "sense of satisfaction in knowing you're helping others get well and stay well" with the right kind of health knowledge.

DATE-FIG TONIC

For the benefit of those who may not have my other book yet, I will repeat the instructions given in it for the things that Frieda has been taking of late.

1–2 pitted dates

1 good-sized fig

6 tbsp. water

Put everything into a blender and mix thoroughly. Drink before bedtime.

APPLE-SPINACH COMBINATION

1 medium-sized apple with skin intact

3 spinach leaves

1 cup water

Blend everything together in a Vita-Mix whole food machine or similar processor for 1 1/2 minutes. *Make fresh each day.* Although this instruction wasn't mentioned in my other juice book, Frieda discovered through her own experimentation that if some of this leftover juice was allowed to sit overnight in the refrigerator, it would not deliver the same rejuvenating effects the next day as freshly made juice would. She attributed this to the strong enzyme activity in the freshly made juice.

GRAPE-RAISIN BLEND

1 cup raisins, packed

1 quart water

*4 cups seedless grapes, washed and stems
    removed*

1 cup ice cubes

Put the raisins and water in a stainless steel saucepan, cover with a lid, and gently simmer on low heat for 40 minutes. Set aside to cool. Then strain juice and discard raisins (or save them for making raisin bread or muffins).

Put the raisin juice in a Vita-Mix machine or equivalent food machine and add the rest of the ingredients. Secure the two-part lid in place and blend for 2 minutes. Divide into two amounts and drink one portion every six hours.

TOOTHACHE

Juice Ice Cubes to Make the Pain Magically Disappear

DESCRIPTION

Substances or objects that convey a sensation of coldness to different parts of the body have frequently been used by doctors to deaden pain when no other kind of anesthetic was available.

Ice Cubes Alleviate Dental Miseries

The worst time to experience a toothache is usually on the weekend or over a 3- or 4-day holiday when dental offices are closed. Here is a handy remedy that will help to reduce much of the excruciating pain until a dentist can be seen to fix the problem for you. However, this treatment requires frequent applications throughout the day because ice cubes tend to quickly melt around body heat.

JUICE CUBES DENTAL PACK

$1/_2$ cup apple cider

$1/_2$ cup carrot juice (canned)

5 sprigs parsley

$1/_4$ tsp. fresh ginger root (grated)

5 drops peppermint oil

Place everything into a Vita-Mix Total Nutrition Center or an equivalent food machine container. Secure in place the two-part lid by locking it under both tabs. Turn the machine on and run for 2 minutes. Pour contents into part of an empty ice-cube tray and put into the freezer until sufficiently firm. Cut one cube in half using a serrated knife. Or else wrap it in a clean cloth and break it into several pieces with a hammer. Put one small piece next to the aching tooth and leave there until melted. Repeat this procedure as often as is necessary until a dentist can be seen.

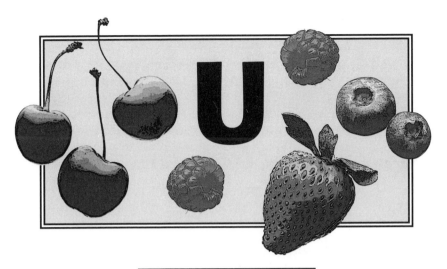

UNDERWEIGHT

(see Malnutrition)

URINARY TRACT INFECTIONS

Ruthless Ex-Dictator Cured Himself with South American Herb Tea

DESCRIPTION

To his enemies, he is a ruthless ex-dictator with plenty of blood on his hands. To the government in Santiago, Chile, he is an immovable object. But to some of his staunchest supporters, he is the man who could be the next president of Chile.

General Augusto Pinochet turned 80 on Saturday, November 25, 1995. He is quite healthy, but still as controversial as ever. There is no talk of retirement from the military he has been in charge of for more than 22 years, with the first 17 also as Chile's ruler.

Pinochet, who ousted a leftist government in 1973 and then governed with an iron fist before leaving the presidential palace in 1990, indicated he enjoys being referred to as "the world's oldest soldier."

The constitution written by Pinochet before he stepped down and permitted the return of democratic elections prevents the civilian president from firing him as commander-in-chief of the Chilean army. It says the post is his to keep until March 1998.

A group of right-wing politicians and prominent businessmen helped to celebrate his birthday with a mammoth banquet in the nation's capital. And at least 80 other dinners around the country were also held that same night as well.

Major Newspaper Revealed Remedy and Other Surprises

There are two major newspapers published in the capital city, Santiago, *El Mercurio* and *La Epoca*. I received by air mail from an American businessman down there who also speaks Spanish a full page torn from the Sunday edition of *El Mercurio*. It contained a lengthy article by the paper's associate editor José Manuel Alvarez.

My American buddy was kind enough to provide a translation of some of the more interesting things the article contained, such as the fact that after Pinochet overthrew President Salvador Allende, a Marxist, in a bloody coup back in 1973, he had an estimated 2,115 political opponents arrested, tortured, and killed in hideous ways. Another 700 or so "disappeared into thin air" after being "politely detained by state security police."

Also, 2,417 people attended Pinochet's main birthday banquet in Santiago, and another 17,610 attending the other 20 dinners held elsewhere throughout Chile. Each person paid the equivalent of $38 for the dinner plus a $100 "donation," which went to the ex-dictator's favorite charity cause, the General Augusto Pinochet Foundation.

But the thing that really caught my attention was the several translated paragraphs dealing with Pinochet's own successful cure for a bad case of urinary tract infection that he had apparently suffered from for some years.

The General's Tea

Pinochet started drinking yerba maté *(Ilex paraguariensis)* sometime in the 1980s, after several Chilean medical doctors gave up on him, saying there was no effective drug therapy for the terrible case of urinary tract infection (UTI) he had somehow managed to contract. Being very displeased with their prognosis, he had one of them brought in for "questioning" by some of his police thugs; the doctor never surfaced again after that.

The remaining physicians who had previously tried to treat him were so alarmed and fearful for their lives that, out of desperation, they consulted with an old *curandero* (folk healer) residing in the slums of west Santiago. This man suggested they give the old boy some yerba maté, which is a national beverage of several South American countries.

Yerba maté is a member of the holly family and is employed as a decorative ornamental in many South American gardens. It and two other members of the holly family are rich in caffeine content: yaupon *(I. vomitoria)* and guayusa *(I. guayusa).* Ordinarily yerba maté was made only from its evergreenlike leaves and twigs. But the old curandero informed the frightened doctors to also include the ripe red berrylike drupes when making the tea.

MAKING MATÉ

1 1/2 tbsp. dried maté leaves, twigs, and berries

1 cup boiling water

Cover the dried plant materials with boiling water and steep for 20 minutes. Then add a dash of lemon juice for flavor and drink with meals twice a day. This is basically how to use maté for clearing up any UTIs.

But as the feature story by editor Alvarez in the *El Mercurio* newspaper pointed out, "the General brews his maté *in style.*" It went on to describe how Pinochet uses a silver-plated gourd called a *culha* in which to steep the plant materials. He then sucks the tea from this fancy gourd with a *bombilla,* a tube about 6 inches long and also made entirely out of silver. At one end is a strainer to keep leaf, twig, and berry particles out of the mouth. He even confided to Alvarez that he liked his maté, which is somewhat bitter to begin with, spike with a dash of lemon juice. "It gives me a brisk rush of exhilaration," the old military tyrant admitted with a wicked gleam in his eye.

Other Health Benefits

The *El Mercurio* article also noted that maté is "an efficacious febrifuge" (for fevers), "wonderful for gastrointestinal disorders" (mostly parasites and heartburn), "pain in the liver" (which I think passes for jaundice), and "diseases of indiscretion" (nothing less than good old syphilis).

I am deeply indebted to Lowell Wickerson for sending me this newspaper clipping, as well for as translating some of the more interesting parts related to my line of research.

UTERINE CANCER

(see Cancer)

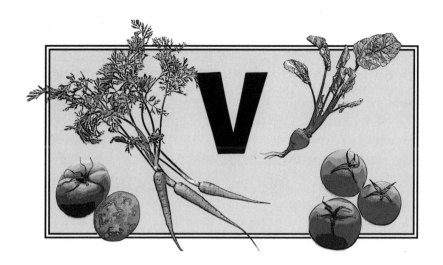

VAGINITIS

(see Yeast Infection)

VARICOSE VEINS

Herbal Trio Makes an Award-Winning Medical Treatment

DESCRIPTION

Oregano is essential in many provincial dishes, ranging from Mediterranean meatballs to the dumplings for an English recipe called Exeter stew to use in diverse French sauces. The Swedes are fond of sprinkling it all over a favorite pea soup, which they almost ritually partake of on Thursdays, for some reason.

Sweet marjoram is a close relative to oregano. It is native to North Africa and southwestern Asia. This is a popular seasoning for sausage mixtures, veal, and fowl.

Both spices are perennial shrubs and can usually grow nearly two feet tall. But in northern Europe, sweet marjoram is unable to tolerate the cold winters and is cultivated as an annual instead. Although prized mainly for their aroma, these plants with their small white flowers are still grown as ornamentals in many European and American gardens.

Dandelion is so pervasive and well known that it begs little need for description. Considered a weed by many people, it commonly grows in waste places, open fields, vacant lots, and hillsides, as well as finding root in well-manicured and kept-up lawns, much to the anguish of homeowners, I might add.

Finding Health Knowledge in Arlington National Cemetery

Twice in 1995 I had occasion to visit Washington, D.C., on matters of business. The first trip was by car across country with two young friends from the small farming community of Henrieville, Utah. Their names were Jeremiah Boger (then age 14) and Stacy Chynoweth (then 16 years of age). The boys and I spent three days there before continuing up to New York City. My second trip occurred alone the following month, toward the end of September. I was back again to interview Utah Congresswoman Enid Waldholtz. (This was before her much-publicized divorce from husband, Joe, whom she later blamed for most of the messy financial scandal she soon became embroiled in.)

Through some other friends, I met a young lady, thirtysomething, who was single, as I am. She worked in the office of California Congressman Sonny Bono (whose ex-wife is Cher), which was located down the hall and around the corner from the Waldholtz office in the sprawling Cannon Office Building. We all went to dinner one night, where the young lady and I became better acquainted.

The next day she gave me a tour of Arlington National Cemetery. I was overwhelmed with what I saw: the neat rows of simple white stones for Civil War dead, stretching to the horizon; the columned, hilltop mansion, once home to Robert E. Lee; the eternal flame by the grave of John F. Kennedy, and the small white cross nearby for his brother Robert. As I accompanied my new friend through the cemetery, I could feel the history behind it, the presence of all the men and women who had endured such horror that we might live in freedom today.

She told me about her varicose vein problems as we walked to the Tomb of the Unknown Soldier. She said her doctor informed her that most of them had been caused by chronic constipation. He had explained to her that her periodic constipation contributed to this in two ways. Her overloaded colon pressed against the veins in her lower abdomen, gradually breaking down the valves located in both the deep femoral and superficial saphenous veins of her legs and permitting a reverse flow of blood. Also, he said, her constant straining at stools increased pressure in these veins and broke the resistance in the blood vessel walls.

An Unknown Remedy at the Unknown Soldier's Tomb

By then we had reached the base of the steps leading up to the tomb itself and the memorial amphitheater located just behind it. Above us, on the plaza fronting the crypt, paced the honor guard from the third U.S. Infantry. I remember how brilliantly the sun gleamed on the visor of his cap.

My friend told me how a friend referred her to someone who taught at Howard University (an African-American school) located in the nation's capital. She made contact with this individual, who was intimately acquainted with herbs. The person suggested an herbal tea made from a trio of common botanicals.

PERFECT THERAPY TEA

1 quart water

2 tbsp. dandelion root

1 tsp. each marjoram and oregano

Boil the water. Add the dandelion root, cover, and simmer on heat for 7 minutes. Uncover and add both spices. Stir well, cover again, and simmer another 3 minutes, then set aside and steep for 20 minutes. Strain and drink 1 cup three times daily on an empty stomach.

As we circled around to the top where the area was roped off, she told me that "within weeks of starting this treatment, much of the stagnant blood that had accumulated in some superficial veins had disappeared; my legs looked better and were no longer painful." She also told me increased walking and wearing looser fitting clothing had helped lower the venous blood pressure in her extremities as well.

By now we were up against the chain separating visitors from the enormous cap of Colorado marble that was the tomb. Everyone around us was hushed in reverent awe; all that could be heard was the click of the sentinel's heels and the slap of his palm on his M-14 rifle. My own reflections went back to the four unknown servicemen interred here, spanning the wars of this century. Each one had served nobly. Each had given his life—better still, his own identity—to a cause he imagined to be greater. And what had they received in return? No thanks or applause, no medals or parades or guest spots on TV talk shows. But this tomb before us stood for things that were important, that lasted forever.

On our way back down my escort also mentioned that she took some vitamin E oil (500 IU), vitamin C (3,000 mg.), bioflavinoids (500 mg.), B-complex (high-potency), zinc (25 mg.), Kyolic garlic (2 capsules daily), and lecithin (2 teaspoons of granules each day).

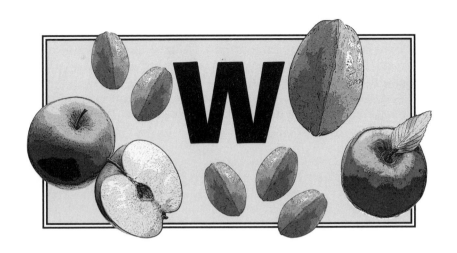

WARTS

A Remedial Measure Passed on During Fat Tuesday's Festival Day

DESCRIPTION

In ancient times Rome, Italy, was the most conspicuous center of carnival activity. The splendor and richness of the festivity that marked its observance were scarcely surpassed anywhere else. When Christianity became the adopted new religion of the empire, numerous elements of heathenism crept into what would eventually become Roman Catholicisn.

Carnivals then took on more of a religious aspect after that. A great deal of merrymaking and festivity began surrounding the last days and hours of the pre-Lenten season. In fact, the word itself can be traced back to the Medieval Latin *carnem levare* or *carnelevarium*, which means to take away or remove meat. Carnivals became the final festivities before the austere 40 days of Lent, during which Catholics, in earlier times, abstained from eating meat.

In France, one of the strongest Catholic countries during the Middle Ages, this festive day was celebrated on the Tuesday (Shrove Tuesday) before Ash Wednesday, which marks the beginning of the Lenten season. It was given the French name Mardi Gras or Fat Tuesday from the custom of devout Catholics of using up all the fats in their homes before Lent began.

Early French settlers to Louisiana brought this celebration with them and expanded its activities somewhat. Ancestors of today's Cajun communities made it their last opportunity for merrymaking and excessive indulgence in food and drink before the solemn season of religious fasting started. And while other cities in the world, such as Rio de Janeiro in Brazil and the cities of Nice and Cologne in France and Germany have similar carnivals, none is so spectacular, outrageous, or famous as the Mardi Gras in New Orleans. It has evolved into an international attraction for that city because of its elaborate parades, masked balls, mock ceremonials, and excessive street dancing, all of which lasts for half a month. The climaxing event is the huge Rex parade on the last night of Mardi Gras.

Wart-B-Gon

It was during one of these riotous January celebrations some years ago that I found myself a part of all that city's craziness. Sleep in any hotel room during normal resting hours was virtually impossible, because of so damned much noise. When I complained about this to one policeman, he looked at me in a funny kind of way and asked with obvious sarcasm, "So what do you want me to do about it, mister—arrest the whole city for disorderly conduct?"

While wandering around the overcrowded downtown district I ducked into one small herb shop for a look around and to collect my sanity. The insulation that this enclosure provided from the racket outside was welcome indeed.

On one of the shelves I noticed a product with a curious name on its label: Wart-B-Gon. It was manufactured by a local outfit. I read the short list of ingredients: alcohol, banana skin, and cashew shells. I held it aloft in my hand and asked the store proprietor if it really worked. "Must do," he said between chews on his plug of tobacco and occasional spits into a nearby metal receptacle on the floor. "I sell out of all that I can get my hands on." He was and still remains in my repertoire of unpleasant memories, the *only* operator of a store selling natural supplements who engaged himself in the filthy habit of chewing and spitting without nary a regard for public opinion.

Imagine my surprise, though, when I looked for the price on it. I was in for sticker shock, if ever there was such a thing. "$19.95! $19.95!" I repeated in loud bewilderment. "You gotta be kidding or something." The guy with the potbelly behind the counter merely shrugged his rounded shoulders and commented, "That's right, mister. Take it or leave it."

Now that I look back on the ridiculous incident, I probably should have paid his outrageous extortion and bought the product as a sample. Instead, I hastily scribbled down the manufacturer's name and address, then put the product back on the shelf and walked out in anger.

Formula Preparation

I paid a visit to the manufacturer, who turned out to be an old gent then in his late seventies. At first he was kind of cagey and hesitant about saying very much concerning his Wart-B-Gon. But after we sat and chatted awhile on other matters, he eventually loosened up enough to the point where he felt comfortable talking about it.

He said the formula had been handed down to him through several generations of grandparents. He said that it worked better than anything he knew of for the removal of warts. When I told him how much the guy in the herb shop was charging, my informant merely rolled his eyes around in his head and kept muttering to himself, "Lordy! Lordy! some folks are greedier than I thought."

Sometime later in our two-hour visit he made it clear he didn't want his name mentioned if I ever decided to use this interview in one of my health books. He also made me promise not to mention his company's name either, for fear of being shut down by the local health department (he kept a number of cats on the premises at all times). Looking into my face and noticing my concern about so many pets inside, he volunteered this humorous explanation: "Leestways, I haven't got a rat problem with them here" (motioning with one bony hand in the direction of some cats).

But, though he gave no precise amounts, he felt confident enough to trust me with at least this much information regarding this special wart-removal preparation. I have synthesized the information he gave me for the reader's benefit.

HOMEMADE WART-B-GON

Some alcohol (preferably "corn likker" or whiskey)

Rotten banana peel ("chopped up good")

Small handful cashew nut shells ("crushed by hammer")

Mix everything together and put in a wide-mouth glass or crockware container (it is strongly advisable to *not* use any kind of metal or plastic for this soaking). When

I tried to get my informant to pinpoint an approximate amount of alcohol, he replied only, "Enough to cover." Set in a cool, dark corner somewhere, cover with a towel, and let it soak for four days. Then strain twice; first through a wire-meshed sieve and then through some clean cotton cloth. Bottle in dark amber glass, if available.

Using an eyedropper, put several drops of this solution on the wart 5 times each day for 10 days or longer. By that time the wart should have disappeared, but continue the use if it hasn't.

WORMS

YEAST INFECTION

Antiseptic Soup Tonic for "Critter" Removal

DESCRIPTION

I remember some years ago meeting a retired country doctor at one of the many health conventions at which I've been a guest speaker during the last two decades. In speaking with this wise old gent on general health matters, I recall a quaint term he used to collectively describe any intestinal parasites or the genus of yeastlike imperfect fungi belonging to the family *Cryptococcaceae,* which induces candidiasis (better known as yeast infection).

The term he used was *critters.* I remarked that I thought the description a little strange coming from a man of medicine such as himself. He snorted and asked why such complicated scientific names always had to be used "which the common lay person doesn't know how to spell worth a darn" anyway. "Isn't it simpler, son," he asked me in his sagacious wisdom, "to just call them 'critters' instead of using high-falutin' words to describe the same things?"

I thought on this for a moment or two before giving my reply in the affirmative. Whereupon he added in jest, "'Sides that, it only shows up the ignorance of the learned more than it does with the unlearned." Discerning my puzzlement as to what he meant by this, my informant went on to philosophize further about what he had just said.

"If a man knows something and can explain it to others in simple language, then he sure as shoot oughta do so. But if he's trying to impress others with his book learning and all by using big, fancy words that nobody can understand, then it shows him up for the fool he is. When dealing with common folks, use the language they're used to speaking and you'll win 'em over, heart and mind." And then, with a nodding motion of his head to move closer in so others wouldn't hear him, he leaned down and whispered in my ear: "Son, it's been my experience that most everybody likes a little piece of ass every now and again, but nobody like a *smart ass!"*

My apologies are offered in advance to any reader whose cultural or moral sensitivity might just have become a little offended at what I've written. But that's how the old boy told it to me 11 years ago and what I wrote down in some notes made of that occasion and filed away until now. I'm just telling it as he stated it to me and trying to preserve a bit of his crusty personality in the hopes that some of his wise, friendly, and kind spirit might penetrate to the reader. In order to adequately do so, I was faced with the necessity of using some of the language he used. I hope, therefore, that any offended readers might find it in their souls to forgive me for what I quoted in the last paragraph, based upon the understanding I've given them.

The Doctor's Soup Remedy

This lovable curmudgeon insisted that he had the "perfect tonic" for what he aptly called "critter removal." "It's as simple as the nose on your face and dimple in your chin," he said with a crackly laugh. And with that he gave me his recipe (or I should say remedy) for expelling worms and getting rid of *Candida albicans.*

Doc's Simple Soup

¹/₂ gallon water

2 large onions, peeled and chopped

1 whole clove garlic, peeled and minced

1 tsp. dried thyme spice

some chicken bones

salt and pepper for taste

Boil the water. Add the chicken bones. Cover and cook for 45 minutes. Uncover and strain broth. Discard the bones. Return the broth to the same pot. Then add the different vegetable spices, cover, and continue cooking on medium heat for another half hour. Set aside to cool. Skim most but not all of the coagulated fat that has accumulated on top, reserving just a small portion for flavor. Reheat enough to melt this fat back into the broth. Then strain it for a second time through a wire sieve, discarding the vegetables.

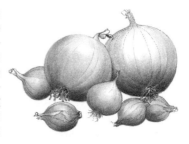

Store in a glass jar with a screw-on metal lid and refrigerate. Reheat enough for one cup and drink twice a day between meals or on an empty stomach for maximum effectiveness. *Note:* In the event you suffer from high blood pressure, omit the salt. Make a fresh batch every couple of days. Besides drinking it, this broth may also be used warm in the form of a vaginal douche to reduce yeast infections.

PRODUCT APPENDIX

A number of different herbs, teas, and tonics are mentioned through-out this text. Many of them can be easily procured from herb shops, natural food stores, or nutrition centers. But sometimes one of these businesses may not be found in places that some readers reside, espe-cially if readers are located in rural or remote settings. Also, a number of juices are recommended here as well that require a good machine to make them, but without discarding the pulpy fiber. Therefore, as a public service to readers of this book, I have included the following fine companies with a brief list of the wonderful products or services they offer. They are all reputable and deserving of consumer trust, otherwise they wouldn't be listed. Readers are encouraged to contact any of them for whatever items they may need to make any of the remedies mentioned herein.

> Vita-Mix Corporation
> 8615 Usher Road
> Cleveland, OH 44138
> 1-800-437-4654

They manufacture the world's best whole food machine. Their Vita-Mix Total Nutrition Center has won numerous awards and acclaim through the years from home economists, nutritionists, doc-tors, and health care providers for being able to liquefy natural foods with everything *intact* and nothing lost. The Rodale Food Laboratory in Emmaus, Pennsylvania, evaluated a number of juicing devices sev-eral years ago and recommended the Vita-Mix unit over all others because of its simplicity, durability, easy cleaning, and affordability. The Vita-Mix Corporation has been around longer than anybody else in the manufacture of food processors, and they make a machine that is world class, tough, and one that utilizes *all* the food and not just certain parts of it as others do. It is the best investment anyone could make for their health's sake!

> Wakunaga of America
> 23501 Madero
> Mission Viejo, CA
> 1-800-421-2998
> 1-800-544-5800 (California only)

The parent company to the American affiliate is Wakunaga Pharmaceutical Company of Hiroshima, Japan, one of Southeast Asia's largest and most respected medicinal products' manufacturer. They developed and market the world's premier-selling aged garlic extract, known globally under the familiar trademark name Kyolic. Hundreds of people I know (including myself, friends, and family) have been using the company's Kyolic EPA (aged garlic extract and fish oil) to help stabilize their serum cholesterol and triglyceride levels. Many other seniors I know of have been taking the company's Kyolic Formulas 105 and 106 to help slow the aging process and give them better qualities of life. Formula 105 is an antioxidant product containing aged garlic extract and vitamins A, C, and E, along with selenium and green tea powder. Formula 106 has in it aged garlic extract, vitamin E, hawthorn berry, and cayenne pepper and is excellent for the functions of the heart, liver, and circulation. Another fairly recent product that has been extensively tested worldwide is Kyo-Ginseng, which combines the antibiotic properties of Kyolic aged garlic extract with the life-giving and longevity-promoting qualities of pure Asian ginseng root extract. Then there is Ginkgo Biloba Plus, a wonderful formula. Several hundred thousand people in the United States and Europe have already benefited from its marvelous effects on the circulatory system. Finally, there is Kyolic aged garlic extract in *liquid* form, which is occasionally mentioned in the text. All these fine products originate with the world leader in garlic research and manufacturing, Wakunaga. It is a name to be fully trusted and is synonymous with quality care the world over.

Pines International, Inc.
P.O. Box 1107
Lawrence, KS 66044
1-800-MY-PINES

These folks are to wheat grass and chlorophyll products what Ford and Chevy are to cars and trucks. The company is owned and operated by American farmers in the nation's heartland, where the best wheat and barley grasses grow. Their products are considered by the natural foods supplement industry to be at the top of their class. No other chlorophyll company in existence can hold a candle to their sterling products, which are available in powder and tablet forms. Numerous lab analyses that have compared Pines with competing lines have also shown the Pines products to be much higher in nutritional content *and fiber* than anything else out there. In fact, more foreign countries buy Pines excellent chlorophyll products in bulk than any other line, simply because the Pines name is revered worldwide for integrity, purity, and nutritional goodness. Pines products repeatedly beat out the competition in test after test and have garnered for the company a lion's share of industry and government awards worldwide. They make wheat grass and barley grass juice extracts; organic beet root juice concentrate; rhubarb juice concentrate; peppermint leaf powder; and an exciting new health drink mix called Mighty Green.

Great American Natural Products & Tea Company
4121 16th Street North
St. Petersburg, FL 33703
1-800-323-4372 / Fax: 1-800-522-6457

Old Amish Herbs & Tea Emporium
4141 Iris Street North
St. Petersburg, FL 33703

The folks who own and operate each of these separate businesses are old-fashioned, very conservative, and highly ethical in all their transactions. Each one in its own way specializes in mail-order botanicals, and both are ideal sources for obtaining top-of-the-line herbal teas, tonics, and similar potions. In addition, each one also carries a wide variety of specially flavored coffees and offers an exotic array of nuts, berries, and seeds. They are the largest distributors of such things in the Southeastern United States. You won't ever find them at any health food industry trade shows or in any ads by them in nationally circulated health magazines. The reason for both is because word-of-mouth satisfaction has been the best-selling factor for each of them worldwide.

John Heinerman, Ph.D.
Anthropological Research Center
P.O. Box 11471
Salt Lake City, UT 84147
1-801-521-8824 (only at 8:30 A.M. Mountain Time)

This is where I can be reached 24 hours a day, 7 days a week, 52 weeks of the year. We carry as a service to consumers the best vitamin E oil available. It is called Rex's Wheat Germ Oil and is used primarily by veterinarians nationwide for their animal patients, but it is of equal benefit for human health needs. It is $65 per quart can.

INDEX